DERVISH YOGA

D1360978

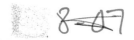

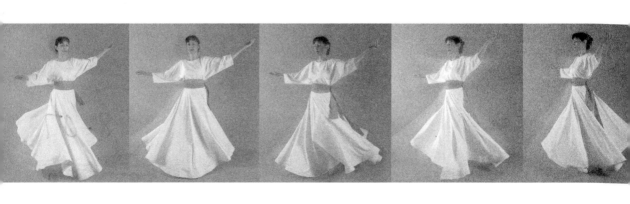

DERVISH YOGA

FOR HEALTH
& LONGEVITY

**SAMADEVA GESTURAL EUPHONY—
THE SEVEN MAJOR ARKANAS**

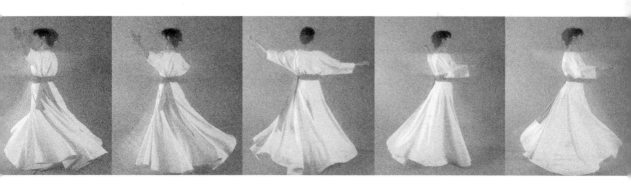

IDRIS LAHORE

ENNEA TESS GRIFFITH · EMMA THYLOCH

TRANSLATED BY MOSES BERGEMAN

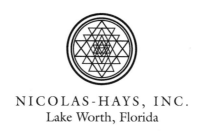

NICOLAS-HAYS, INC.
Lake Worth, Florida

8-07   10.17

First published in 2007 by
Nicolas-Hays, Inc.
P. O. Box 540206
Lake Worth, FL 33454-0206
www.nicolashays.com
Distributed to the trade by
Red Wheel/Weiser, LLC
65 Parker St., Unit 7
Newburyport, MA 01950-4600
www.redwheelweiser.com

Library of Congress Cataloging-in-Publication Data available on request.
Cover and interior photography by Pierre Christoph
Cover design and interior layout by Kathryn Sky-Peck
Typeset in ITC Century

Printed in the United States of America
VG

12   11   10   09   08   07
6 5 4 3 2 1
The paper used in this publication meets the minimum requirements of the
American National Standard for Information Sciences—Permanence of Paper for
Printed Library Materials Z39.48–1992 (R1997).

CONTENTS

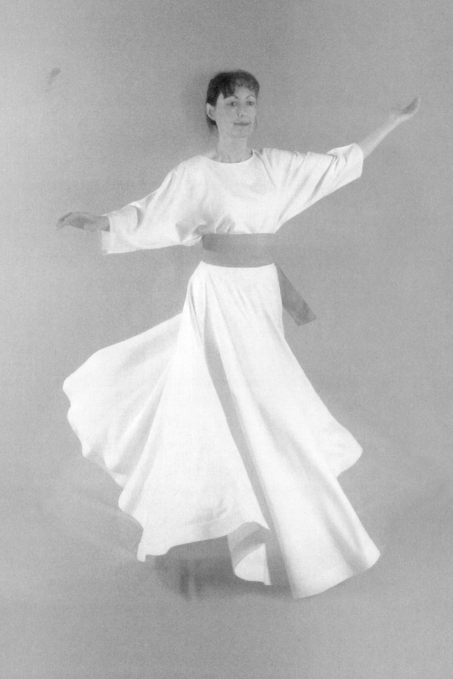

PREFACE

Ennea Tess Griffith

I founded the Free University of Samadeva at the impulse of Idris Lahore. My goal was to offer both knowledge and practical techniques for improving our physical well-being and furthering our inner development. To realize this goal, I have integrated practical techniques from the East, such as Zen, yoga, and qi gong, with methods developed in the West during recent decades, like stretching, relaxation, sophrology, and eurhythmy. In this way, the wisdom of the East and the science of the West have found, in the work of the Free University of Samadeva, their most harmonious expression.

As a psycho-corporal method, Samadeva Gestural Euphony is one of the pearls of this work. With the valuable aid of my colleagues, especially Emma Thyloch, I worked tirelessly at perfecting Samadeva Gestural Euphony. My contacts with doctors, therapists, yoga teachers, specialists in the field of sacred dances, and dervishes have been a source of continual enrichment and have helped me perfect the method.

Idris Lahore, a remarkable man, travelled across the globe, from China to Spanish Andalusia, passing through Tibet and India, Arabia and Persia, Palestine, and Egypt. Wandering dervish among the dervishes, he assimilated both theoretical and practical knowledge from his Sufi

1

friends, especially in the field of medicine, which he practiced himself for many years. In this way he was able to
adapt the most effective techniques of the ancient Masters
of Wisdom, whose legacy was passed on to the dervishes,
to our Western medicine. These learned and erudite men
taught at the great Islamic universities of the Middle Ages,
which at the time of their decline were replaced by our
Western institutions with their experimental science and
systematic research.

Idris Lahore, "my friend and Teacher" (to quote from a
well-known contemporary song), while reserving his traditional medical knowledge for his friends in the medical
field, taught me everything issuing from this knowledge
that belongs to the paramedical realm, which in former
times played an essential role in the art of healing—specifically, the art of music, the spoken word, and song, the art
of gesture, movement, and dance, and the art of nutrition,
essences, and fragrances.

Thus the traditional component of Samadeva Gestural
Euphony has its roots in the most ancient teachings of the
Eastern schools of wisdom, the schools that gave birth to
most currents of thought from antiquity to the present day.
Beyond the yogic, Sufi, Taoist, and Zen philosophical
schools developed over the course of history, Samadeva
Gestural Euphony permits us to rediscover their common
original source, from which I retained the most important
and relevant methods.

Their effectiveness, recognized scientifically, is connected to a profound knowledge, which gives us a system that can be used both preventatively and curatively, promoting a long and healthy life.

During weekly classes, known as "model sessions" (see pages 131–132), or during training seminars and weekends, everyone can experience the harmony which, above and beyond the many different methods, characterizes Samadeva Gestural Euphony. At once a philosophy and a practical method, Samadeva Gestural Euphony is also a way of life.

The seven major Arkanas are a fundamental part of Gestural Euphony, the psycho-corporal branch of Samadeva, which itself also includes eight further branches (see the Nine Branches of Samadeva, pages 179–182) that can be discovered at the Free University of Samadeva, particularly during its annual congress.

I sincerely hope that the seven major Arkanas presented here bring you inner calm and joy and help you toward the realization of your highest goals.

"O Sun, rise and awaken, the atoms are dancing,

The souls, bodiless, are dancing, are dancing with joy,

He who sees that the heavens and firmament are dancing,

Into his ear shall I tell him whither leads the dance."

RUMI, *Rubaiyat,* IX

INTRODUCTION

Idris Lahore

The seven major Arkanas of Samadeva Gestural Euphony are simple, yet extraordinarily revitalizing. They are addressed to everyone between the ages of three and ninety-nine. In the past, in their secret brotherhoods, the dervishes called them "the exercises of rejuvenation."

Indeed, they fortify the body, relaxing it and filling it with a new energy. In addition, they restore the psyche to a state of equilibrium and regenerate the mind, increasing its vivacity and slowing the aging process. Practicing Samadeva, you will have the energy you need to live fully and calmly. The people around you, your spouse, parents, children, friends, and colleagues, will equally benefit. You will be physically fit and internally calm, and your intellectual capacities will be heightened. All of your functions will be stimulated and harmonised.

Resembling such techniques as yoga, tai chi, relaxation, eurhythmy, and light gymnastics, Samadeva mobilizes all of your physical, emotional, and mental resources, allowing you to adapt effectively to the situations of your daily life.

Everyone wants health and a long life—more specifically, a long life in good health! How can we stay young? Are the secret of eternal youth, the secret of immortality of the alchemists and Taoists legend or are they reality? Samadeva

Gestural Euphony teaches us techniques that permit us to live in good health and grow old without aging, in other words to stay young in mind, heart, and body.

In the ancient Schools of Wisdom, the Masters transmitted techniques and methods for physical, emotional, intellectual, and spiritual health. Samadeva Gestural Euphony is the adaptation of the most effective among these, particularly the seven major Arkanas, for the men and women of today. They are based on the knowledge transmitted by the Sarman Schools, a spiritual dervish brotherhood located in the Middle East.

FROM HEALTH TO PERSONAL DEVELOPMENT

Idris Lahore

The range of Samadeva Gestural Euphony extends from simple physical exercises to psychology, health, and metaphysics. Through the variety of its psycho-corporal techniques, its action upon our physical and psychological health and, further, its interest in the context of personal development, can be explained.

Our experience with patients and with people in good health (but with illnesses to come!) has shown us that there are two possible sources of pathogens. The first, which we share with organic and mineral life on earth (humans, animals, plants, air, water, and the earth itself), is connected to the world surrounding us and all of the more or less violent harmful factors ensuing from it.

Verbal or chemical factors, psychological pressure or atmospheric pollution, dietary or intellectual poisons—all of these influences are harmful to our health and lead to the appearance of specific pathologies, sometimes visibly and spontaneously, and sometimes more gradually and insidiously. All of the body's systems—nervous, endocrine, cardiovascular, respiratory, or digestive—may be affected.

The second possible source of pathogens is specific to man, since he alone possesses consciousness. We will not linger on the question of the origin of consciousness (is it innate or acquired, conditioned or unconditioned?) but content ourselves with observing that it is a non-negligible aspect of human life, since it conditions a considerable part of man's thoughts, emotions, and actions. It is at the origin of all of our existential questions with their entire range of possible fears and dissatisfactions, whose psychosomatic consequences are today no longer a mystery to anyone.

As a psycho-corporal method for restoring our equilibrium and health, Samadeva Gestural Euphony helps us relativize external pathogenic influences, rendering us more adaptable, stronger, more balanced, and more resistant. Its second action is aimed at the inner source of pathogens, responding to the question of how I can master, rather than be dominated by, the destructive effects of fear, anxiety, depression, nervousness, and psychosomatic problems, from stomach ulcers and migraines to asthma, high blood-pressure, spasmophilia, and so on, and culminating in much more serious pathologies such as cancer.

psycho-corporal method for restoring equilibrium and health

Learn to master... or rather become "master of oneself" and one's inner mechanisms, rather than remaining their slave, at their mercy: these are the propositions and effects of Samadeva Gestural Euphony.

learn to become "master of oneself" and one's inner mechanisms

This leads us to consider in greater detail the two types of influences upon man: external influences (such as other people, nature, and events), and internal influences (the way we react to the preceding—our thoughts, emotions, feelings, moods, and attitudes).

The possible action upon external influences harmful to our health is a matter of ecology and sociology, understood in their broadest sense. The possible action upon internal influences is connected to a work of understanding and conscientious personal action according to our level of understanding. This is not limited to simple intellectual understanding, but also implies physical and emotional understanding, literal savoir faire.

The techniques of Samadeva Gestural Euphony are to be considered in this context. Based on the most diverse psycho-corporal practices, Samadeva Gestural Euphony integrates an essential cognitive element, placing it beyond simple physical and psychological health techniques into a holistic perspective, and touching the very essence of human nature in the manner of Zen, yoga, or eurhythmy.

an essential cognitive dimension touching the very essence of man's nature

The starting point of Samadeva Gestural Euphony is the threefold nature of man. Consisting of a physical, material body, man arose from the evolution of minerals, plants, and animals on earth, and this binds him to the material world and renders him subject to its laws, namely of birth, growth, degeneration, and disappearance or death. The higher element is what we call "consciousness." Between the two lies the third element, the psyche, the object of study of psychology. Religions call this the "soul," the scene of all the emotional, sentimental, and intellectual trials and tribulations of man. Samadeva Gestural Euphony extends its study of the psychological domain to the study of consciousness, as well as the relation of both to the

man's threefold nature

physical body. It must be realized, however, that this ana-lytic-pedagogical division is by no means opposed to the non-tripartite (more familiarly, non-dualistic) reality of the world, nor to the essential perception of the underlying oneness behind this division.

Man's challenge is to go beyond the animality still fully present in him, developing his consciousness which, as yet, exists only partially. The psyche serves the role of interme-diary between the two, strongly stamped with the mark of animality in its lower parts and with consciousness in its higher parts.

The terrible fact of the matter is that man still seems to be, to a great extent, at the level of the animal, and human-ity as a whole is very far from using all available resources for its possible evolution. Nonetheless, for certain people who begin to acquire a certain knowledge and understand-ing and then undertake a specific "work," it becomes possi-ble to evolve toward higher and more harmonious states of consciousness and being.

humanity is very far from using all resources for its possible evolution

From the standpoint of his possible evolution, it is essential to understand that a part of man is animal, and that this animal nature is responsible for the majority of his thoughts, emotions, and actions. This fact represents the first limitation, the second being the conditioning of his family, education, society, and religion. Understanding this is the beginning of an accurate perception of man's situa-tion in the world, which is anything but free. Nevertheless, freedom becomes possible when, after having understood

freedom becomes possible when man, after becoming conscious of his limitations and conditioning, undertakes a work of transformation

his limitations and conditioning, he undertakes a work of transformation.

This is the proposition of a possible line of work that has Samadeva Gestural Euphony as its starting point. In other words, the acquisition of what people think they already have, freedom, is possible but only physical, emotional, and intellectual "work" can lead to its attainment. Freedom is not a characteristic of man, but a possible acquisition.

freedom is not a characteristic of man, but a possible acquisition

But why is man more animal than genuinely human? And why is he influenced so much by the conditioning of his education?

Man is sometimes described as a "three-brained" being. The first brain governs his physical body and instinctive life. It has a tendency to aggressiveness with an excessively developed sense of property (greed, territoriality, and so on). This is the oldest brain, the "reptilian brain," the brain of birds, snakes, crocodiles, and other reptiles.

the "reptilian brain" governs the physical body and instinctive life

The second brain, termed "limbic," governs his emotional life, with all of its moods, desires, feelings, and pursuit of pleasure. More evolved than the first, physical brain, it was initially the point of departure for the sense of smell, subsequently developing and extending to the entire emotional realm. It nevertheless remains an old, animal brain.

the "limbic brain" governs the emotional life

The third brain, the "neocortex," is the brain of the intellectual center. More recent from an evolutionary standpoint, it is at the origin of man's possibility of raising himself above animality by developing the faculty of thought that is

the "neocortex," the brain of our intellectual center

characteristic of humanity. Culture, technology, and the arts have their source in this brain.

Given the fact that two thirds of the human brain is still imprinted with animality, and that the most recent part is not particularly developed, it shouldn't surprise anyone that man and humanity are, still today, dominated by animal attitudes. Some of these are more or less connected to the instinctive life, such as aggressiveness, the sexual instinct, competition, or the instincts of property, greed, and egocentrism; others are more tied to the emotional life, such as the desire to dominate, fear, jealousy, arrogance, pride, and vanity. The fact is that the cause of individual unhappiness, and of collective tragedies, can be found in the persistence of attitudes having their origin in the animal world, from the dramas and tragedies of passion (jealousy, sex) to ethnic or economic wars (property instinct, greed).

the cause of individual and collective suffering is to be found in the persistence of attitudes originating in the animal world

The question is: how can we avoid the negative side effects arising from the very real presence of the animal instincts? What is the appropriate place of the animal nature in man? How can we place it at the service of the evolution of the higher, with the awareness that the intellectual center, our thought alone, is insufficient? In any case, it has been insufficient up until now…

But before we search for answers to these questions, let us first examine the other forms of conditioning to which man living in society is subject. Conditioning is just as limiting a factor as the animal instincts we described above. If we are aware of this, we can understand human behavior and all its paradoxes and contradictions, for example, the opposition between our real possibilities and desires, realism and demands, thoughts and emotions, good intentions and results, prejudices and reality, etc.

The three categories of conditioning are directly connected to the three brains: reflexive conditioning to the physical brain, pleasure-pain conditioning to the emotional brain, and imitative conditioning to the intellectual brain. In the same way that we cannot dismiss our animal reality, a part of our conditioning is obviously necessary for our social life, and a certain part of it even for our survival.

Reflexive conditioning of the physical body consists in the association of a natural need to artificial external stimuli not directly connected to it. For example, hunger is a natural need, and the sound of a bell summoning us to the dining room is an external stimulus—this sound induces salivation and the sensation of hunger, which Pavlov described so well in his experiments with dogs.

Pleasure-pain conditioning is more tied to a seeking of something than to an elicited reflex: seeking reward (pleasure) or desiring to avoid punishment (pain). Finally, imitative conditioning is connected to the necessity of socialization and the need for identification. A significant part of our education is based on this process, beginning with personal hygiene and extending to more elaborate customs and manners within the whole range of social attitudes, physical, emotional, or intellectual. In this connection, the most subtle and harmful conditioning results from the fact

understanding human behavior with its paradoxes and contradictions

three categories of conditioning

reflexive conditioning

pleasure-pain conditioning

imitative conditioning

that we are forced to believe a certain number of things. A typical example is national chauvinism, being brought up to be proud to be French, American, or Russian, etc. This means that very many of our attitudes, opinions, beliefs, and thoughts have simply been inculcated in us by our education; we have been literally indoctrinated, and the limitations arising from our conditioning are just as powerful as our natural, instinctive limitations.

The prisons of our animal instincts, and the innumerable prisons of our conditioning—this is what Samadeva Gestural Euphony proposes that we become conscious of in several different ways.

becoming aware of our many prisons

His ignorance of these mechanisms is not only the principal reason for man's inner alienation and interpersonal difficulties, but also, as we will see, for his problems of health and personal development.

The paradox is that these mechanisms are processes of both adaptation to life and deterioration of life at the same time. The question thus arises: how can we preserve and improve the processes of adaptation and eliminate or diminish the effects of the processes of deterioration?

how to preserve and improve the processes of adaptation and eliminate or diminish the effects of the processes of deterioration?

This is where Samadeva Gestural Euphony comes in. We know that the accumulation of negative emotions and stress disrupts the sympathetic and parasympathetic nervous systems, causing chain reactions in the endocrine, digestive, cardiovascular, or respiratory systems, with consequences for the secretion of cortisol and endorphins. All of this takes place under the influence of neurotransmitters or synaptic transmitters, with the result that the harmonizing capacities of our bodily and psychological mechanisms are diminished.

The exercises of Samadeva Gestural Euphony act upon the musculature, giving it both tone and flexibility—our muscles and tendons work more effectively, with more resistance and a greater endurance, resulting in improved coordination. This brings with it a diminishing of chronic pains and psychosomatic problems. In addition, the exercises allow us to experience such forgotten physical sensations as inner calm and peace, contributing to a positive reprogramming of the realm of our sensations; the diencephalon is calmed rather than being adversely affected by the stress of our everyday life. We feel relaxed; anxiety and nervousness are replaced by calm and serenity. Thanks to these positive sensations, the participant rediscovers a positive perception of life, he learns to better master himself and better accept his environment, which is no longer perceived as stressful or harmful. This leads him to experience a new joy of living and increased self-confidence. Greater self-knowledge and knowledge of other people allow him to integrate himself more positively into his life, and this has even further positive effects on his health.

action of the exercises of Samadeva Gestural Euphony

experience such forgotten physical sensations as inner calm and peace

THE HARMONIZATION
OF THE CHAKRAS

Idris Lahore

W̓e are not only composed of a physical organism with its various cells, organs, and systems, but also of an energetic structure, consisting of energetic centers and pathways, whose proper functioning is just as important for our health, well-being, development, and physical, emotional, intellectual, and spiritual equilibrium as the proper functioning of these cells, organs, and physical systems.

energetic centers

Our energetic organism comprises very many energetic centers, the most important of which are the seven chakras as they are described by the Hindu yogis. "Chakra" means "wheel" or "moving circle." The most well-known are the seven principal chakras, each divided, at the next level, into seven sub-chakras. Certain traditions, like that of the dervishes, specify three hundred further chakras, the most important of which are to be found on the chest, on each side of the heart chakra, and on the abdomen, on each side of the sexual chakra; in addition, two chakras are located on the palms of the hands and two on the soles of the feet.

seven energetic centers containing the organism's forces of life

The seven principal chakras are the energetic centers containing the organism's forces of life. They are located close to the cerebro-spinal system and serve simultaneously as the memories, energetic accumulators, and brains of all the energies that enable the human organism to live. Each of these seven chakras memorizes, accumulates, governs, and distributes specific energies. As a system, they govern not only our physical body, but also our emotional "body" and thought "body," and beyond these, our spiritual "body" and systemic "body" (in connection with all of our relationships, of any nature, with people living or dead, and with objects, animals, plants, places, events, and so on). We can consider these energetic centers as transforming the most subtle energies into nerve impulses and cellular or hormonal energy for our physical body.

These energies are distributed from the chakras along more than three hundred thousand energetic pathways known as "nadis." The nature of each chakra corresponds exactly, not only to human nature in general, but also to the completely specific personality of each individual.

When someone cultivates emotions, thoughts, words, and actions that correspond to human nature, the chakras function harmoniously and supply his organism with energy of this same harmonious quality. In contrast, when someone cultivates thoughts, emotions, words, or attitudes that are contrary to human nature—that is to say, conflictual—the energies connected to the chakras tend to be dispersed outside of his organism, giving rise to a deficit of energy in his thoughts and feelings as well as his actions, and leading to disruptions or disconnections in the circulation of energies along the energetic pathways (nadis).

The chakras are also in direct relationship with man's higher consciousness, his inner wisdom or subconscious

each of the seven chakras memorizes, accumulates, governs, and distributes specific energies

the chakras transform the most subtle energies into nerve impulses and cellular or hormonal energy for the physical body

energetic pathways or meridians

equilibrium and perturbation of the chakras

essence. Their proper functioning is essential to his possibility of entering into contact with his own inner wisdom and for his whole organism—body, soul, and spirit—to function euphonically, that is to say, harmoniously.

Although they have a privileged relationship with the endocrine glands, directly influencing growth as well as most of our physiological functions via the nervous system and blood circulation, the chakras also have a specific effect upon our emotions, feelings, and thought schemas, and this influence is reciprocal.

Muladhara, the first chakra or "root chakra," connects us with our roots—our family, ancestors, country, race, culture, education, social milieu, and religion. It is the chakra of belonging and of the survival instinct. It is the measure of our identification with and gratitude toward those to whom we owe everything we are, and often everything we possess.

This base chakra is located in the region of the genital organs, at the lower extremity of the vertebral column; it is connected to the kidneys and adrenal glands. It has a particular relation with the emotion of fear. Its activity is very pronounced during the first seven years of man's life, during which he is especially interested in everything relating to his growth. He needs to be fed and taken care of in order to survive, since during this phase of his life, the child is not yet capable of fulfilling his needs on his own. This chakra acts upon the skeleton, excretory organs, lymphatic system, external sexual organs, and ovaries and testicles, which produce the hormones estrogen and testosterone. It directs the

direct relationship with higher consciousness, one's inner wisdom or essence

*FIRST CHAKRA
MULADHARA
ROOT CHAKRA*

energies of the arms and legs. It also acts upon the sense of smell and is connected to the element earth. Also called the "moving center," this first chakra directs all of our external movements. These external movements are not innate but must all be acquired through learning.

The first chakra functions harmoniously when we cultivate the love of nature, when we recognize its beauty and protect it through actions that are respectful of the air, water, earth, plants, and animals; it is fortified when we breathe pure air and nourish ourselves with organically—or biodynamically—grown foods.

It is balanced when we recognize with gratitude each thing that has been passed on to us by our parents and ancestors, by our teachers and the citizens of our country, without demanding or regretting whatever they may not have given us.

This chakra is reinforced when we manifest our gratitude through acts of respect, kindness, and service toward the people belonging to the different groups and communities to which we have belonged or still belong.

The first chakra is weakened when we fail to cultivate the love of nature, when we do not recognize its beauty and instead pollute the air, water, earth, plants, and animals; likewise when we breathe polluted air and eat degraded and chemical foods.

It is perturbed when we deny what has been passed on to us by our parents and ancestors, our teachers and the citizens of our country, demanding and feeling entitled to whatever they have not given us. This chakra becomes unbalanced when we are disrespectful of other people, particularly when our behavior is egocentric and we fail to cultivate a relationship of love, affection, friendship, and respect with the living or dead members of the different groups to which we have belonged or still belong.

matter and survival

The first chakra is above all the chakra of survival. In adults, it is balanced when we are correctly rooted in the earth and in nature. This is the chakra that gives us the feeling of being in good relationship with our environment, and particularly with the material world. When it is perturbed, we are lacking in confidence, and we become overly greedy and sometimes violent. We may also have the impression of being a stranger in our own environment. We have problems with money or material possessions and we are unable to find our rhythm in life.

Everything we have said concerning this first chakra does not imply that we are completely chained to everything we have received from the different groups to which we have belonged; we are connected to these groups by the ties of life, and provided we preserve the respect for these ties, we are free to evolve in other societal groups or to create another family beyond our original family.

The fact that we belong, as human beings, to humanity as a whole also means that we cannot consider our own family, race, religion, political party, social class, and all the opinions and beliefs that are bound up with them, to be superior to those of people belonging to different groups; they are simply different opinions and different beliefs. In the same way, if the opinions, beliefs, or attitudes of the groups we belong to are opposed to a greater humanism or humanitarianism, we have to be able to integrate this humanism, otherwise our first chakra is once again weakened.

Swathisthana, the second chakra, is also called the sexual chakra. Whereas the first chakra is responsible for our relationship with an ensemble of individuals and groups, and with superhuman forces such as the forces of nature, the second chakra is the chakra of our inter-individual relationships, namely our sexual and love relationships, friendships, and professional relationships. This chakra is reinforced between the ages of seven and fourteen. During this period, our sensual and sexual perception develops simultaneously with our creativity and imagination.

SECOND CHAKRA
SWATHISTHANA
SEXUAL CHAKRA

sensuality, sexuality, creativity

It is especially associated with the ovaries in women and the testicles and prostate gland in men. Its element is water, and it has a direct relationship with all of our body's liquids (blood, urine, lymph, and so on). It acts upon the adrenal glands (producers of cortisone and adrenaline) as well as upon the sense of taste.

the second chakra related to the element water

This chakra is the organism's accumulator of energies, which it subsequently redistributes to all the other chakras. It is the great accumulator of all the vital energies.

When our relationships are governed by love, friendship, respect, kindness, and tolerance, this chakra functions in a balanced way. In contrast, our interpersonal conflicts disrupt its functioning. This is particularly true of all forms of

equilibrium and harmony of the second chakra

competition and of the desire to dominate or control other people. Competition, jealousy, opposition, resentment, and personal hostility weaken this chakra, as do all forms of sexual disorders and abuse. The state of balance or unbalance of this chakra likewise conditions our relationship to money and possessions in all their forms. It is disrupted by our dependencies, whether they are of an affective, sexual, dietary, or other nature.

perturbation and weakening
of the second chakra

Someone who is well-anchored in this chakra has a good awareness of his body, in which he feels comfortable and at home. He accepts and respects himself. He is capable of leading a creative life and entering into a mature relationship with those around him. He develops a healthy sexuality which manifests itself through pleasure and joy. The false education children receive about sexuality leads to a disorder of this chakra, and later on to disorders of all kinds—the individual has much difficulty being in contact with his or her own body and having a healthy enjoyment of the pleasures of life. People who are strongly afflicted with problems in this chakra have difficulty expressing their own creativity; there exists in them a refusal of their own body, and thus a nonacceptance of themselves which often leads to auto-immune diseases. The repression of sensuality or sexuality leads to a repression of the vital force.

energy of relationships

Manipura, the third chakra or solar plexus chakra, is particularly fortified between the ages of fourteen and twenty-one, the period during which the desire to control and desire for power emerge, and also the desire to realize one's

THIRD CHAKRA
MANIPURA
SOLAR PLEXUS CHAKRA

dreams. The third chakra is the chakra of the individual's relationship to himself; this is the chakra of the love, respect, and esteem we cultivate toward ourselves.

It is the chakra of self-confidence and the localization of our inner force. It is from this chakra that we take on responsibilities and fulfill our engagements. It is the source of our intuition, and allows us to establish or recognize our own limits.

personal power and transformation

Someone who is balanced in this chakra has a natural esteem of himself and an ability to live life serenely, enjoying it completely naturally.

equilibrium and harmony of the third chakra

When this chakra is well-developed, we will be able to realize our dreams; when it is in disorder, our dreams remain simply dreams, or else turn into nightmares.

This chakra acts upon the sense of sight. It is also involved with digestion in the stomach, the transformation and purification of blood in the spleen, the secretion of digestive juices and production of insulin in the pancreas, the production of bile and transformation of carbohydrates into glycogen, or energy, in the liver, and the storage of bile in the gall bladder; it is connected not only to digestion and assimilation in our physical body, but also to the digestion and assimilation of our emotions, thoughts, and the events of our lives.

When this chakra is perturbed, we either have a tendency to gorge ourselves with too many things that we are unable to digest, or we are unable to absorb anything at all, and this is true for our emotions and external impressions just as much as for our material food.

perturbation and weakening of the third chakra

The energy of the third chakra is weakened when we do not recognize our own limits, when we allow other people to be disrespectful of us, when we use other people to our own ends, trying to attract their attention or approval, or when we seek to manipulate them to our own advantage.

When the energy of this chakra is disrupted, we are prevented from expressing ourselves, either because we have not got our feet solidly on the ground, or because we remain too attached, too imprisoned by our thought schemas and everything in us that is old, incapable of opening ourselves to the new life of every moment. When it is unbalanced, this chakra leads us to be untrue to ourselves, to our opinions, our thoughts, our promises, our honor, and our word.

perturbation and
weakening of the
third chakra

The perturbation of this chakra also gives rise to a tendency to worry, anger, or complaining, as well as a tendency to surround ourselves with people who worry and complain. The illnesses resulting from a perturbation of this chakra include stomach ulcers, problems assimilating sugar, and the majority of digestive problems.

When it is disrupted, this chakra also leads to egocentrism and vanity, a strategy for hiding our deep-seated doubts about our own worth, and thus a sense of inferiority. Other people, in contrast, may be very introverted, incapable of correctly expressing themselves outwardly.

the third chakra related to
the element fire

The element of this chakra is fire; an excess of fire leads to violence and a lack of it to depression, as if one were extinguished, "burned out."

Anahata, the fourth chakra, is the heart chakra, the chakra of love—particularly the love of other people—and of compassion and forgiveness. It is the chakra responsible for the balance of our whole organism and of the chakras among each other. This is where love of ourselves is integrated with love of other people, and also where it is possible to overcome all our negative emotions, particularly resentment and hostility, which are replaced by unconditional forgiveness, permitting us to overcome all our past sufferings and respect the destiny of every person whatsoever.

It is associated with the heart, lungs, and thymus; it governs a considerable part of the immune system, and its element is air. It acts upon the sense of touch.

In this chakra, the vital energy is anchored through the respiration. It is the chakra of both joy and of sadness—joy when it is balanced, and sadness when it is perturbed. Smiling and laughing have an extremely powerful effect upon this chakra, and as smiling and laughing also stimulate the thymus, they have an effect on the immune system as well. One of the most important treatments for immune diseases is to learn to laugh and, more than anything, to smile. We only need to picture to ourselves the blissful smile of lovers in order to realize that their whole emotional, bodily, and even intellectual organisms are stimulated. This is also the smile of those who meditate, and the smile of the Buddha.

FOURTH CHAKRA
ANAHATA
HEART CHAKRA

harmony and love

the fourth chakra related to the element air

equilibrium and perturbation of the fourth chakra

emotional energy

the heart chakra connects the three lower chakras with the three higher chakras

FIFTH CHAKRA
VISSHUDA
THROAT CHAKRA

voluntary energy

related to the
element ether

expression and
communication

perturbation and
weakening of the fifth
chakra

Visshuda, the fifth chakra, that of the larynx, is above all the chakra of expression, will, decisions, and choices. It governs the energies in the arms and hands. It acts on growth and metabolism and on the prolongation of the spinal cord, the medulla oblongata.

The element of this chakra is space or ether, and it is connected to the sense of hearing.

Its balance is ensured when we sincerely and honestly express our own words, choices, and decisions. It is also the chakra of self-mastery.

The perturbation of this chakra gives rise to a poor functioning of the glands—hypothyroidism or hyperthyroidism, for example; we then either have a lazy metabolism, resulting in weight problems, or become overly restless and hyperactive. It is disrupted when we allow other people to control our own needs or desires. It is weakened by lying and strengthened by honesty and uprightness. The only form of submission that can balance this chakra is submission to higher forces, the forces of the soul, the spirit, the Origin, Absolute, or Divine; at this moment it can function in synergy and harmony with our understanding, will, and higher principles.

The perturbation of the fifth chakra also leads to difficulties expressing ourselves with words and communicating with other people, to difficulties expressing our truest, most deep-seated thoughts and our most genuine emotions.

When this chakra is balanced, we are far-removed from illusions and ready-made thoughts, and we express ourselves much more genuinely, free from dogmas and rigid thought schemas.

equilibrium and harmony of the fifth chakra

The tradition teaches us that close to this chakra, another chakra, Latifa Lalana, secretes a sweet liquid, the elixir of immortality, the divine nectar amrita which, according to certain dervishes and yogis, permits a person to survive without eating or drinking.

Latifa Lalana

Ajna, the sixth chakra or third eye, is located in the middle of the forehead. It is the chakra of discernment, of rational and logical intelligence, but also of inspiration. In this chakra, the force of the heart can join to the intelligence of the mind. It is the center of a higher form of creativity, in very close relationship with the soul and essence, as well as with the universe.

SIXTH CHAKRA
AJNA
THIRD EYE CHAKRA

energy of thought, inspiration

It is in direct relationship with the pituitary, which we can consider to be the gland that directs all the other glands and all the other bodily functions. It directs the rhythmic systems of the body, particularly the sleep-waking rhythm, but also the adaptation to changes of the seasons. It is connected to the optic nerve and the olfactory bulb.

When this chakra is perturbed by excessively dualistic, logical, rational thought, it limits the impulses from the heart. This kind of dogmatic, rigid, critical, judgmental thought is often closed to new ideas.

perturbation and weakening of the sixth chakra

When we are too attached to the material aspects of life, this chakra functions in disequilibrium; this in turn renders us incapable of seeing the truth, since we are connected exclusively with material truth which, for our essence, is incomplete and fragmentary.

Disturbances of this chakra are often accompanied by problems with vision and headaches.

equilibrium and harmony of the sixth chakra

When it is functioning harmoniously, it helps us overcome rationalism and the limitations of the logical mind—our imagination and creativity can then take flight. It also permits us to enter into contact with other worlds, to understand the laws of synchronicity, and to perceive what is hidden behind appearances.

SEVENTH CHAKRA SAHASRARA CROWN CHAKRA

Sahasrara, the seventh chakra or "crown chakra," is located on top of the head, in the area of the fontanel. It is the chakra of our relationship to the Higher, to the Origin, the Absolute, the Divine, the chakra of the spiritual path, of liberation, awakening, or inner realization, beyond all duality and all separativity. It is through this chakra that we can enter into contact with what is higher in ourselves, with our essence.

spirituality

It governs the cortex and nervous system, and it is in relationship with the pineal gland.

equilibrium and harmony of the seventh chakra

Its state of equilibrium permits us to understand that our earthly life is a passage during which our spiritual evolution is possible. Life is the occasion for this evolution, which is its principal goal. This chakra permits us to understand higher principles and to confide ourselves in these principles, recognizing all sources of spiritual guidance.

It is the location of true conscience, transcending all forms of acquired moral conscience (which themselves have their seat in the first, root chakra). It permits us to truly live in the present, beyond the limitations of the past and future.

According to tradition, the energy present in the first chakra is capable of ascending along the nadis, or energetic pathways, of the vertebral column, attaining the seventh chakra and permitting man to realize the consummation of his potentialities.

spiritual energy

•   •   •

NOTE: All of the chakras are connected with each other, and in each chakra we can find specific aspects of all the others.

FIRST CHAKRA element earth	family and ancestral energy	matter and survival *"each part is a part of the whole (all is one)"*
SECOND CHAKRA element water	energy of relationship	sensuality and sexuality *"respect of other people, of diversity, and of differences"*
THIRD CHAKRA element fire	personal energy	personal power and transformation *"respect of one's own individual nature with its own destiny"*
FOURTH CHAKRA element air	emotional energy	harmony and love *"wherever two or three are gathered, a higher Force is present"*
FIFTH CHAKRA element space or ether	voluntary energy	expression and communication *"integration of personal will in the higher will"*
SIXTH CHAKRA	energy of thought	inspiration *"seeker of truth"*
SEVENTH CHAKRA	spiritual energy	spirituality *"the Presence of the Force of the Origin"*

THE SEVEN MAJOR ARKANAS

PHYSICAL & PSYCHOLOGICAL BENEFITS

Ennea Tess Griffith & Idris Lahore

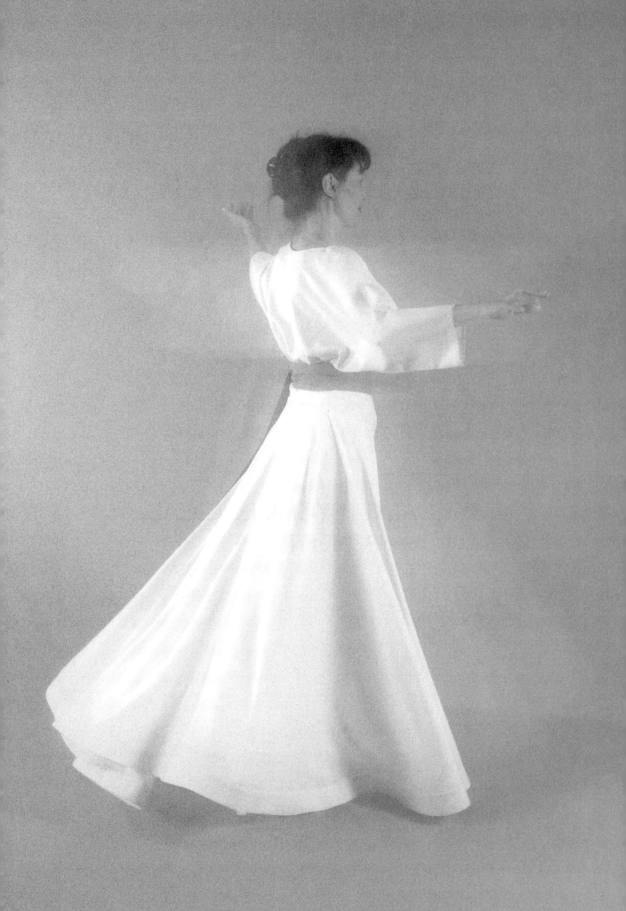

HEALTH

Genuine health is the state of equilibrium between our physical functions and organs and our emotional and intellectual functions. Our everyday life, with its entire range of experiences and difficulties (all of our illnesses and worries, for example) causes us to lose, with each day, that fragile equilibrium which is health, with the sad result that most people in our day age prematurely. Good sleep and a healthy diet no longer suffice for us to regain our equilibrium; we need the help of health specialists and methods of reharmonization and healing.

Samadeva Gestural Euphony, with its extraordinary rejuvenating effects, is addressed to precisely this situation. Practicing the Arkanas of Gestural Euphony, you will see that they are not just physical exercises, but have the most profound and positive effects on your emotions and moods as well as on your concentration and memory.

PHYSICAL AND PSYCHOLOGICAL WELL-BEING

The Masters of the past were well aware of the role played by our muscles, as it has been rediscovered by modern science. Our muscles are the connecting link between our body and psyche; our psychological tensions are inscribed in our muscles and, conversely, our physical tensions give rise to psychological fatigue and restlessness. This interdependence permits us to understand the importance of good muscle tone. By practicing the movements and positions of Samadeva Gestural Euphony, we harmonize the functioning of our muscles, resulting in sufficient muscle tone for activity and eliminating unnecessary tensions for relaxation. This results not only in physical well-being, but in psychological equilibrium as well.

The eminently positive psychological effect of regular practice can also be explained by the fact that the Arkanas act upon the different parts of the brain, which are thus better oxygenated. They improve the action of substances such as hormones and neurotransmitters, whose role is precisely to transmit messages of equilibrium and proper functioning to all the organs, down to the body's very smallest cells.

Psychological equilibrium is characterized by a clear mind, confidence, and optimism, and a feeling of youth and freshness. It is also characterized by an excellent resistance in the face of stress, difficulties, and worries, accompanied by a good, regenerative sleep. It manifests itself especially through a contagious joy of living.

THE NEUROPHYSIOLOGY OF ATTENTION

The focalization of attention depends physiologically on the specific part of the cerebral cortex associated with the stimulation of significant interest in a particular subject. In the context of Samadeva Gestural Euphony, this is further accentuated by acoustic and musical stimuli. The concentration elicited by practicing the exercises leads to a hyperfocalization, reducing the field of perceptions and eliminating those that are not useful. An improvement in attention and, as a consequence, an improvement in memory can be verified.

Hyperventilation following certain exercises increases the diffusion of cortical inhibition, particularly due to the diminution of plasmatic CO_2, with a depressant effect on the highest termination of the ascending reticular activator system. This leads to a depression of the excitability of the cortical neurons. Thus the biochemical, circulatory, metabolic, and bioelectric effects act in synergy, improving concentration.

Since the postures, movements, and dances are unaccustomed and sometimes momentarily unnatural, they lead to a destabilization of the posterior labyrinth, with a significant excitation of the vestibular centers. This phenomenon stimulates concentration, which may then focalize to an even greater degree due to the action of the cutaneous proprioceptors and exteroceptors resulting from the movements in space.

GENERAL POSITIVE EFFECTS

Substantial effects can be verified in the venous, arterial, and lymphatic systems, with an improvement in blood circulation to the brain (resulting in better memory and concentration) and to the extremities (hands, legs, and feet), as well as a harmonization of arterial tension and stimulation of the cardiac muscle, improvement of physical resistance, purification of the lungs and improved oxygenation of the blood resulting from respiratory techniques and movements, increased flexibility of the vertebral column and joints (with each session, the body becomes more flexible, agile, and resistant), stimulation of the digestive organs through self-massage of the abdomen, stimulation of the kidneys, skin, and excretory organs, regulation of the male and female endocrine systems, harmonization of the sexual function, reinforcement of the immune system, emotional and psychological harmonization and appeasement, and development of intuition, creativity, and inspiration.

PHYSICAL, EMOTIONAL, AND MENTAL HARMONIZATION

The manner of inhalation and exhalation leads very rapidly to an improvement of equilibrium and reinforcement of the nervous system, with obvious effects upon nervous tensions and insomnia.

Beginning with the nervous system, the effects of the seven major Arkanas subsequently extend to the locomotor apparatus (muscles, joints, and tendons), the endocrine system, and the digestive, respiratory, and urogenital systems.

Practicing the Arkanas, the entire organism is stimulated, the psyche calmed, and the mind clarified.

Because all the senses are functioning better, the energetic centers or chakras (see pages 17–31 and page 51) are able to better absorb the energies outside the body. The harmonization of the internal energies—the physical, emotional, and intellectual energies—then takes place completely naturally. Man and woman, innerly balanced, can thus live in harmony with other people and with their environment.

Samadeva Gestural Euphony becomes the simplest, most enjoyable, and most effective way of acquiring and preserving health, vitality, harmony, and youth.

THE SEVEN MAJOR ARKANAS

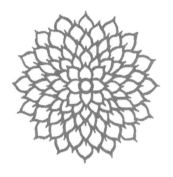

A GUIDE TO PRACTICING
THE EXERCISES

Emma Thyloch & Ennea Tess Griffith

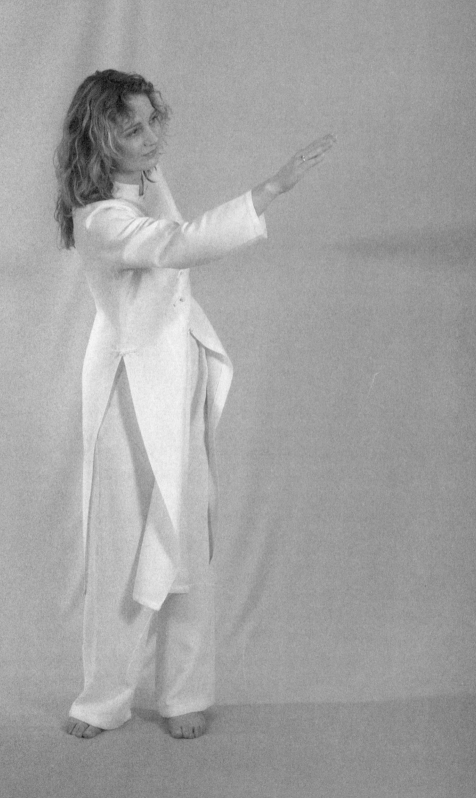

HOW TO BEGIN PRACTICE

Practice should be progressive: learn one Arkana after the other until you have reached the seventh. Increase the length of the exercises only gradually (ten minutes are enough for a beginner and for regular daily practice). Practicing in this way, you will make rapid progress and perform the Arkanas better and better with time.

This may require a few efforts at the outset, but with time the movements will become simple and flowing. Then you will have mastered the Arkanas, and you will be left with the pleasure of doing them and of reaping their extraordinary benefits of regeneration, revitalization, rejuvenation, and health.

You can practice the Arkanas at any time, and because of their diversity, you can simply choose the ones you like most according to the time and place.

The movements and postures of the Arkanas are by no means fixed and rigid; each person may adapt them according to his or her individual body type. The speed with which you do them may also differ according to your temperament or your goal—that is, whether you prefer to be stimulated or calmed. Nevertheless, the ideal situation is to attend a Samadeva Gestural Euphony training session with an instructor, or to participate in an introductory course with an instructor at the Free University of Samadeva.

A FEW HELPFUL TIPS

Some tips in order to facilitate the practice of Samadeva Gestural Euphony: wear loose clothing that does not hinder your breathing, blood circulation, or the movements. When possible, remove your glasses, watch, necklaces, or bracelets.

Avoid practicing the Arkanas with a full stomach.

For certain Arkanas, it is best to have a wool carpet or large bath mat. It is preferable to practice in a well-ventilated room, and to open a window if necessary, but making sure that the room remains at a comfortable temperature.

Never force things; in order not to injure yourself, do every movement gently. If you are tired after doing the Arkanas, this means you have either practiced too much or that you are about to come down with an illness.

If joint pain, or another form of pain, is awakened at the beginning of the movements, practice more gently, and if the pain persists, consult a therapist. In fact, everything that reveals itself is the sign of a problem that ought to be treated. A persistent physical pain is the sign of a physical problem, but it may also be the sign of incorrect or excessive practice.

PRACTICING WITH SUITABLE MUSIC

Samadeva Gestural Euphony is also a "dance therapy" and music therapy, since it is always practiced to the accompaniment of music. Certain exercises culminate in therapeutic choreography that makes use of the dynamizing effects of music. It then serves as a non-verbal group psychotherapy which does not seek conscious oral expression, but relies instead on the curative powers of the unconscious, the voluntary and conscious element being our presence to our postures and movements in the "here and now."

The unconscious is no longer considered exclusively as the Freudian realm of our shadows and repressions, but rather as a positive process capable of leading to the resolution of all our problems, provided we approach them, in the manner of a Milton Erickson, with the right attitude and with the appropriate corporal techniques; and these techniques are not just a matter of physical exercises, but also entail profound and positive effects upon our emotions and moods, upon our concentration and memory as well.

THE SEVEN MAJOR ARKANAS

THE CASCADING FOUNTAIN

REEDS IN THE WIND

HIP DANCE

SUN SALUTATION

STRETCHING OF THE JOY OF LIFE

SPARKS OF FIRE

DANCE OF THE PLANETS

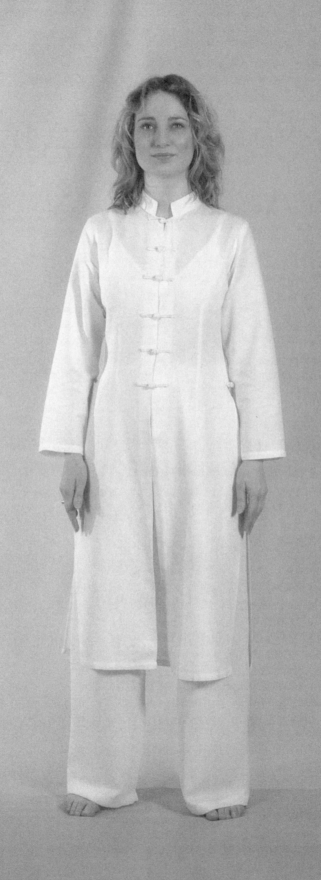

THE FUNDAMENTAL POSITION

We adopt the fundamental position before practicing each Arkana. It is a basic position throughout the course of the exercises. Stand upright, your feet in line with your hips. Bend your knees slightly. Tilt your hips forward slightly, so that your upper body is straight. Place your entire body weight on the front part of your feet, as if your heels were just barely touching the ground. Look straight ahead. Breathe calmly from your abdomen and relax your stomach and lower abdomen. Do not forget to relax your shoulders.

This straight, upright position, with your body weight distributed over both feet, rebalances your vertebral column. Your head and brain are then well-supplied with blood and the different parts of your brain better connected. Your concentration is improved, your breathing deeper and calmer, and your endocrine glands are stimulated.

When practiced with great attention and consciousness, the postures have a beneficial effect on stability, and the movements a beneficial effect on balance. The movements are not hurried, and never forced. They flow gently and gracefully.

THE IMPORTANCE OF BREATHING

Breathing plays a very important role, and once we have mastered the exercises, very precise instructions are given for each Arkana. But at the beginning, it is best to breathe freely while we are learning the movements and postures, making sure that we do not hold our breath—our breathing must flow. The respiratory exercises are added at a later stage. Until then, practice the basic breathing rhythm, in which we exhale for twice as long as we inhale, always pausing for two seconds between inhalation and exhalation.

When we concentrate on our inhalation and exhalation, this leads very quickly to an improvement in our balance and a strengthening of our nervous system, with subsequent effects on possible nervous tensions or insomnia.

Breathing is of primordial importance; your life began with your first breath and will end when you exhale for the last time. All things begin and all things end with respiration. Respiration is at once the most individual and most interpersonal act there is. Each of us needs to breathe in order to remain alive, and at the same time, the air we inhale and exhale is the same for everybody; whether we like it or not, we are connected to everyone around us by the air we breathe.

THE HARMONIZATION OF THE CHAKRAS

Like yoga, Taoism, or the Kabbalah, the dervish science of Samadeva Gestural Euphony has a perfect knowledge of the functioning of the physical body as well as of the "energetic body," consisting of energetic centers and pathways.

The energetic centers or chakras (see pages 17–31) are located along the vertebral column and govern not only the nervous and endocrine systems, but all the other systems and functions of the body as well. From a spiritual point of view, they are said to capture the universal energies (which have different names according to the different traditions: qi in the Chinese, Nafa in the dervish, ruh in the Sufi, prana in the Ayurvedic, and kundalini in the yogic tradition), after which they are able to circulate throughout the entire organism along the different energetic pathways known as meridians in Chinese medicine, Silsilla in dervish medicine, and nadis in Ayurvedic medicine.

The seven major Arkanas have a harmonizing action upon the "energetic body." They progress from the first Arkana, The Cascading Fountain (pages 55–59), which activates and awakens the chakras (thus preparing our physical and energetic bodies for the following Arkanas), to the seventh Arkana, the Sama (pages 101–107), which sets all the centers and energetic pathways in motion.

"And my soul also is a cascading fountain."

Nietzsche, *Thus Spake Zarathustra*

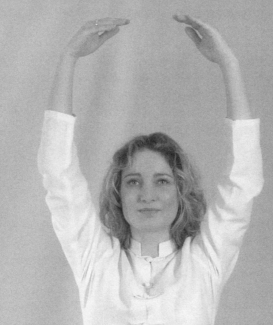

ARKANA 1

CHAKRA LALEH
THE CASCADING FOUNTAIN

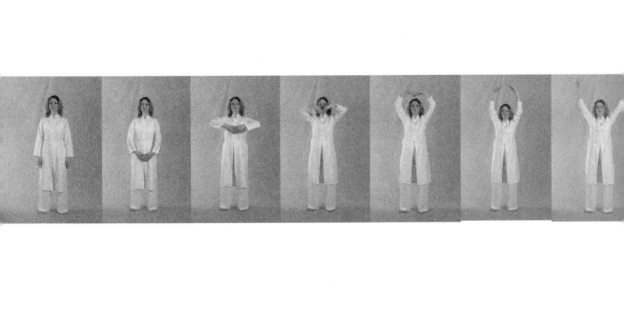

THE CASCADING FOUNTAIN

*This Arkana acts principally upon the nervous system
and regulates the energies.*

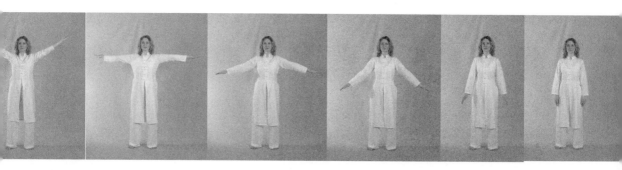

The first Arkana, "The Cascading Fountain," serves as a "warm up," as it were,
awakening and activating our energetic centers or chakras; our physical and
energetic bodies are then prepared for the following Arkanas.

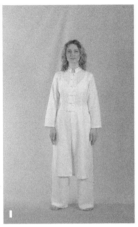 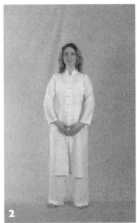 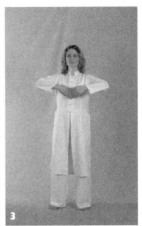 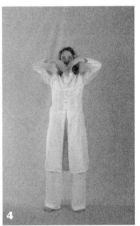

1) Begin in the fundamental position (page 49), your arms relaxed along the length of your body.

2) Join your hands together, forming a triangle at the base of your torso.

3) Pass your hands over all the chakras (for their locations, see the following pages).

4) After passing over the sixth chakra, your hands naturally pivot...

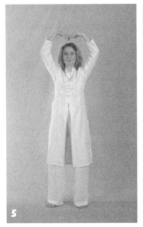 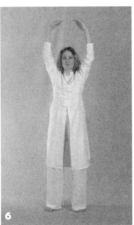 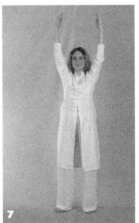 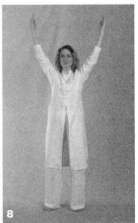

5) ... before arriving at the seventh chakra, at the top of the head.

6–8) Continue ascending, then separate your hands in a semicircular motion, like a cascading fountain.

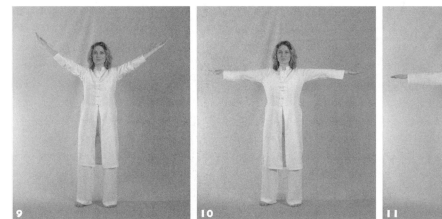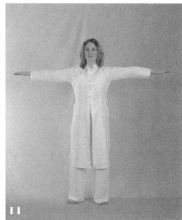

9–10) Lower your arms until they are horizontal, the palms of your hands facing the sky, and always remaining attentive to your bodily sensations.

11) Turn your palms to the ground...

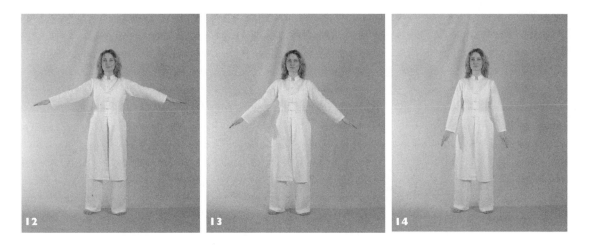

12–14) ... and continue descending until your arms are once again along the length of your body.

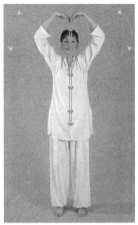 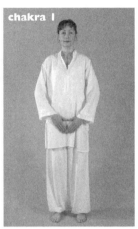 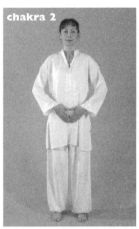 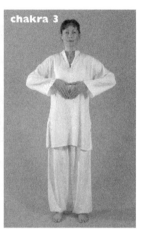

After this initial passage over all of the chakras, during which the movement should be steady and continuous, repeat the passage once again, but pausing this time for ten seconds, your hands forming a triangle, over the first chakra, before passing over the other chakras. Then during the following passage, pause over the second chakra, and continue in this way up to the seventh and final chakra.

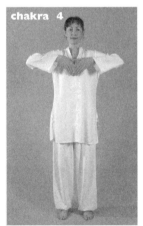 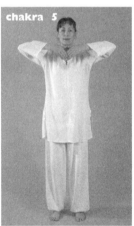 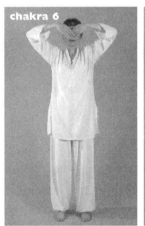 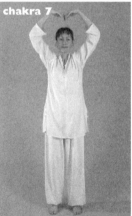

For the pause at the seventh chakra, at the top of your head, just lightly touch this chakra with your fingertips after joining both hands together (see photograph).

After these seven passages, pass over all of the chakras two more times, steadily and continuously, just as in the initial passage.

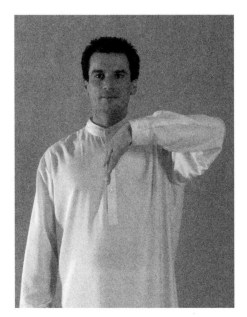

The final, concluding sequence is a triad of "affirmation, negation, and reconciliation." During the "affirmation," your right arm alone passes over all of the chakras, with a steady and continuous motion, your left arm remaining along the side of your body. The position of your ascending right hand is shown (as if in a mirror) in the photograph on the left. Then continue with the "negation," in which your left arm alone passes over all of the chakras, and conclude with the "reconciliation," both arms passing over the chakras as in the initial passage.

Do the movements slowly, remaining attentive to the sensations of your body. When thoughts arise, simply let them pass and return to the sensations of your body.

Total length of the exercise: about 3 minutes

In summary: the complete exercise consists of the initial passage (pages 56–57) **plus** seven consecutive passages, pausing for ten seconds over the first chakra during the first passage, pausing over the second chakra during the second passage, and so on until the seventh chakra (see photos on page 58) **plus** the initial passage two more times **plus** the triad "affirmation, negation, reconciliation" described above.

*"Like the reed that sways in the wind,
and straightens itself ever again."*

Idris Lahore, "Arane, O Arane"

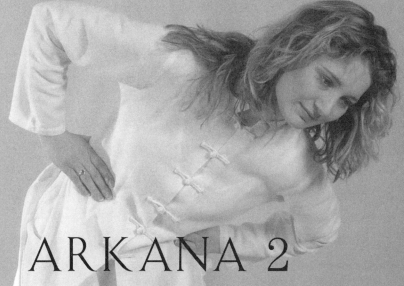

ARKANA 2

NADABRAMA
REEDS IN THE WIND

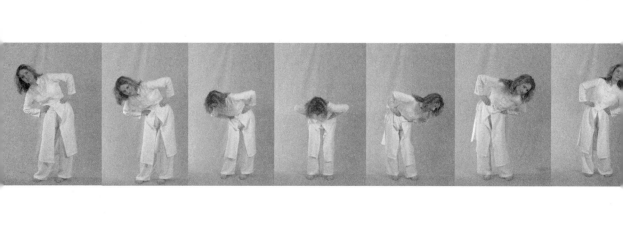

REEDS IN THE WIND

This Arkana acts principally upon the digestive system and vertebral column.

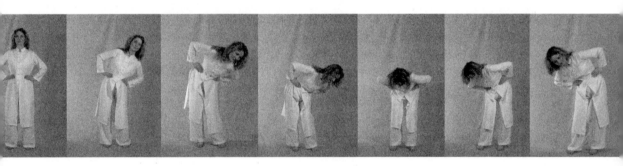

"Movement is the source of all things. Every movement is the manifestation of
an archetype, of a will of the Origin."

ADJITA DJEEMASH

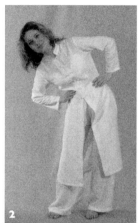 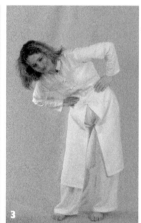 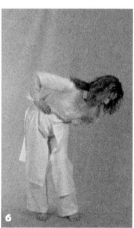 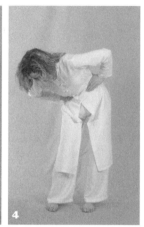

1) Begin in the fundamental position, then place your hands on your hips.

2) Tilt your waist to the left, your shoulders and head to the right.

3–4) Rotate your torso from right to left, your head remaining in line with your vertebral column …

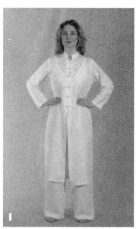 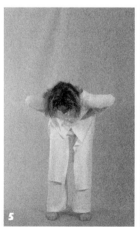 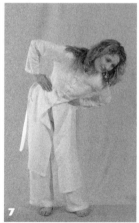 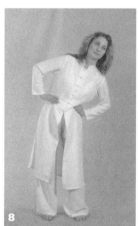

5–6) During the rotation, when your torso is facing forward, in a horizontal position, tilt your waist to the right, your shoulders and head to the left.

7–8) Continue the rotating movement until you have returned to the vertical position. Repeat the complete rotation two more times.

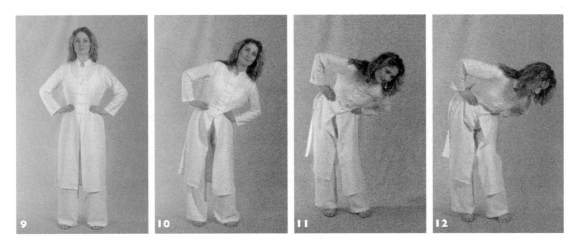

9–16) Pause for a moment in the vertical position, then do three rotations in the other direction: waist to the right, head and shoulders to the left...

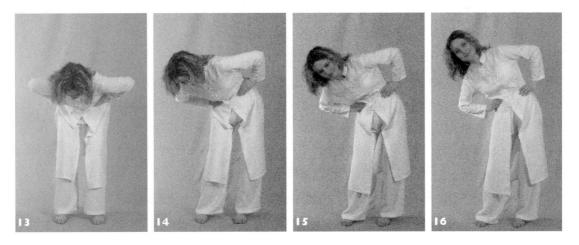

The movement should be continuous, regular, and flowing, like reeds in the wind.

*"Only in the dance do I know how to speak
the parable of the highest things."*

Nietzsche, *Thus Spake Zarathustra*

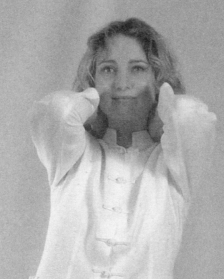

ARKANA 3

NADASAMA
HIP DANCE

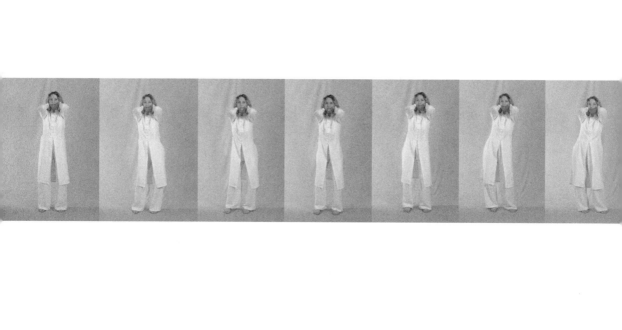

HIP DANCE

*This Arkana acts principally upon the nervous system
and regulates the energies.*

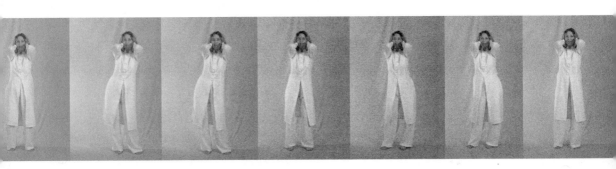

"What we cannot discover through our body, we cannot discover
in any other place in the world."
IDRIS LAHORE, "The Silence of the Body"

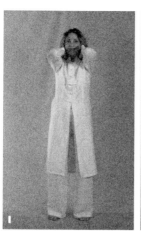 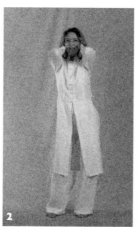 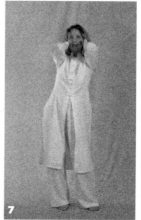 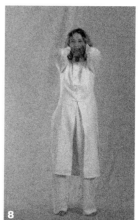

1) Begin in the fundamental position. Interlace your fingers behind your neck. Place your feet firmly on the ground, and keep your head as vertical as possible, looking straight ahead.

2–4) Tilt your waist to the left, then rotate your hips toward the rear.

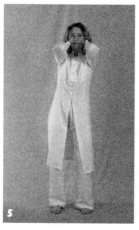 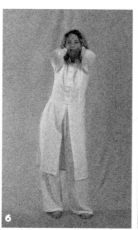 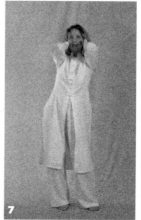 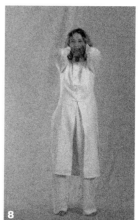

5–8) Now tilt your waist to the right, and rotate your hips toward the front. Your torso is straight, yet flexible. Make sure your upper body remains as immobile as possible; it is your hips that do the dancing.

Repeat three times, then return to the fundamental position.

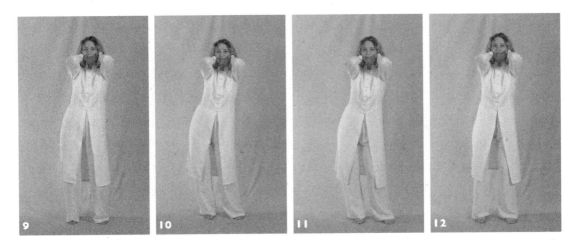

9–16) Now do three rotations in the opposite direction: waist to the right, hips rotate toward the rear; waist to the left, hips rotate toward the front...

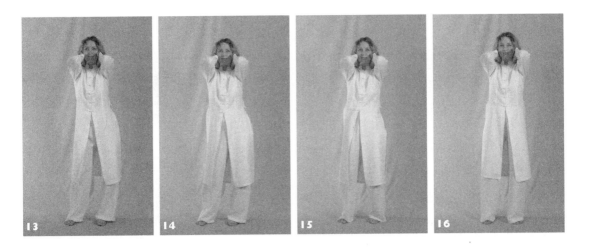

When practiced regularly, this exercise corrects the position of your hips and lumbar region.

"Man, a being who one day acquired the vertical position,
like a bridge between heaven and earth..."

IDRIS LAHORE

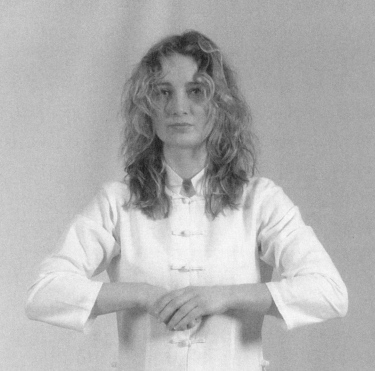

ARKANA 4

AHURAMAZDA
SUN SALUTATION

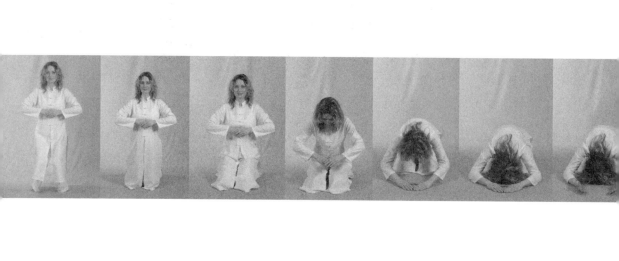

SUN SALUTATION

This Arkana is the exercise for health par excellence. It acts upon all the bodily functions, especially the heart and blood circulation and the joints.

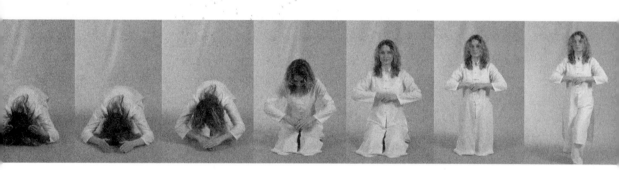

"The seven major Arkanas are built upon man's evolution over the ages. Through them we can inwardly rediscover the path of the human soul across time and the evolution of worlds."

IDRIS LAHORE

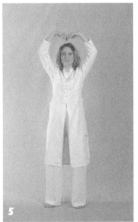
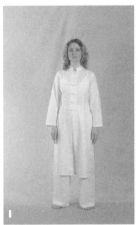
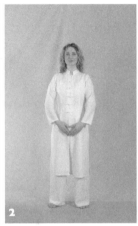
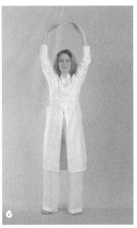
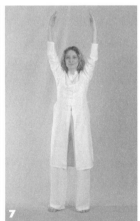
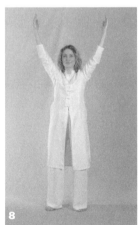
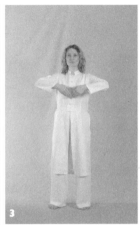
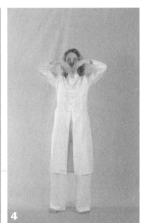

1) Begin in the fundamental position, your arms relaxed along the length of your body.

2) Join your hands together, forming a triangle at the base of your torso.

3) Pass your hands over all of the chakras.

4) After passing over the sixth chakra, your hands naturally pivot…

5) … before arriving at the seventh chakra, at the top of your head.

6–8) Continue ascending, then separate your hands in a semicircular motion, like a cascading fountain.

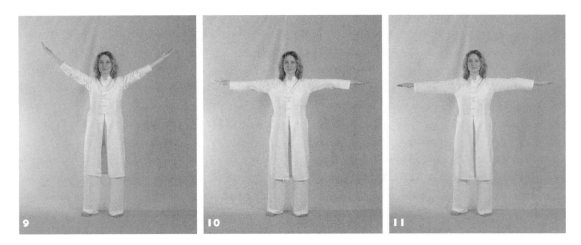

9–10) Lower your arms until they are horizontal, the palms of your hands facing the sky.

11) Turn your palms to the ground...

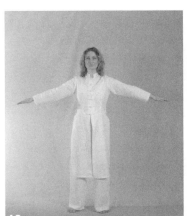 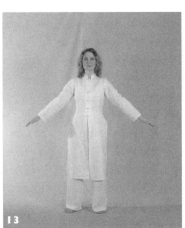 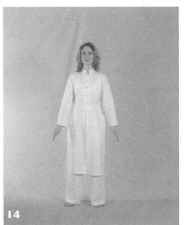

12–14) ... and continue descending until your arms are once again along the length of your body.

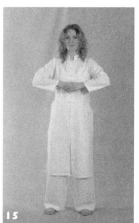 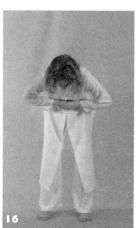 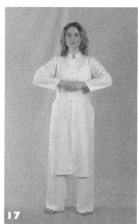 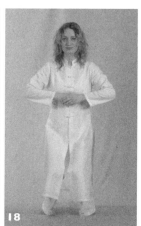

15) Join your hands together in front of your solar plexus, holding your left thumb in your right hand.

16–17) Bow forward, then return again to the upright position.

18–19) Now descend to your knees…

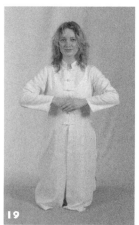 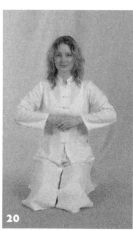 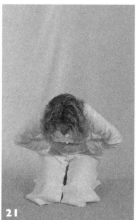 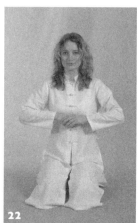

20) …and continue descending until you are sitting on your heels.

21–23) Bow again in salutation, and return to the upright posture.

The movement is calm, light, and flowing.

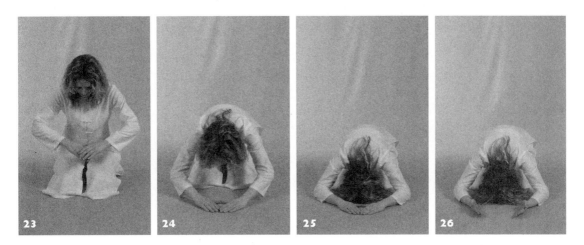

23) Bow forward a third time.

24) Continue bowing and place your hands upon the ground, forming a triangle.

25) Place your forehead on the ground, prostrating yourself.

26) Turn the palms of your hands upward, separating your hands.

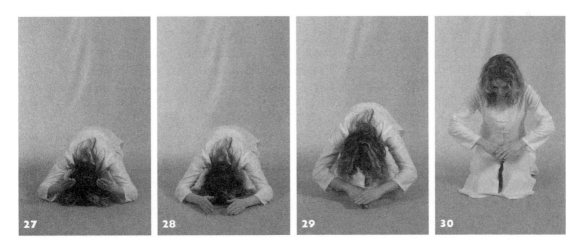

27–28) Lifting your forearms, raise your hands toward the sky, then place them once again upon the ground in the triangle position.

29–30) Straighten yourself, again placing your left thumb in your right hand.

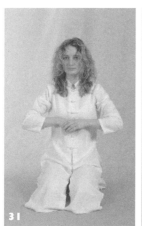
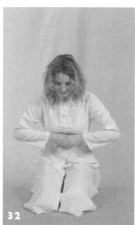
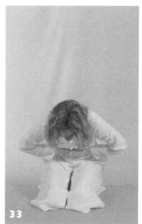
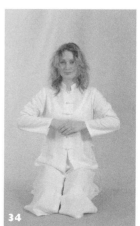

31) You are once again sitting on your heels, and your torso is straight.

32–34) Bow again in salutation and straighten yourself.

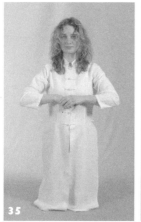
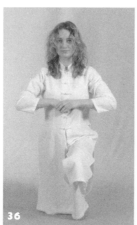
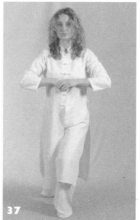
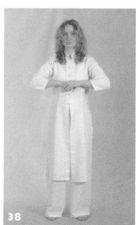

35) Raise yourself onto your knees.

36–37) Stand up, using your left foot.

38) You have returned to the upright position, and your hands are still together, your left thumb in your right hand.

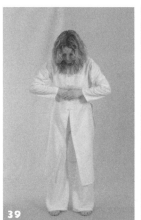 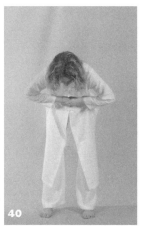 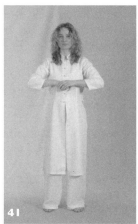 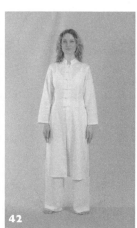

39–40) Bow once again in salutation.

41–42) After straightening yourself, allow your arms to descend along the length of your body.

Each of the movements flows continuously into the next.

Important: Never force things, do everything gently. People who have joint pain or difficulty kneeling may replace the kneeling movements with similar movements in the upright position. Instead of prostrating themselves, they may place their hands and forehead upon an imaginary horizontal plane extending from their chest.

The sun salutation has been practiced since the dawn of time in all the Mystery Schools, sometimes in slightly varying forms. It has always been considered to be the foundation of all spiritual practice.

It associates the body with the mind, and since each movement gives rise to a feeling or emotion, the heart also participates.

It is the fundamental exercise of the body, heart, and mind for attaining inner peace.

THE SUN SALUTATION:
THE BENEFICIAL EFFECTS OF ITS DIFFERENT POSTURES

The upright, straight position, with our body weight well-distributed over both feet, rebalances our vertebral column, with a beneficial effect upon blood flow to our brain as well as the interconnection among its different parts. Our concentration improves, and our breathing becomes deeper and calmer; our endocrine glands are also stimulated.

When we bow in the upright position, the muscles of our lower back, thighs, and calves are stretched. The blood rises to the upper part of our torso. Our digestive organs—stomach, liver, gall bladder, pancreas, and intestines—are stimulated.

The kneeling movements of this Arkana render the joints of our arms and legs and our back more flexible. Blood flow to our head increases, which in turn improves the functioning of our lungs, bronchial tubes, eyes, nose, and ears. These movements also have an excellent effect upon high blood pressure.

The movement of prostration has a very particular effect upon our psychosomatic state. It balances us, harmonizing our sympathetic and parasympathetic nervous systems, and permits us to overcome our egocentrism.

THE SUN SALUTATION: AN EXPRESSION OF GRATITUDE FOR THE DIFFERENT KINGDOMS OF NATURE

When he stands upright, man is who he truly is: a being who one day acquired the vertical position, like a bridge between heaven and earth. When he bows, he is like the plant, like the reed swaying in the wind. When he is kneeling, on all fours, he is like the animal. And when he prostrates himself, he returns to the mineral kingdom. Thus over the course of the sun salutation, man passes once again through all the stages of his evolution. He remembers that he is composed of the different natural kingdoms, which find in him both their union and their culmination. This Arkana is also the expression of his gratitude for these different kingdoms.

At the same time, the sun salutation teaches us that each creature occupies a specific place in the creation, a place that corresponds to its level. It is said that even the angels have a specific posture for expressing their love of God! Man alone is capable of adopting any of these postures; he is free to choose between that of the animal, the plant, or the dust and—one day—to learn that of the angel. Legend also tells us that whoever practices the sun salutation is accompanied by two angels, his guardian angel and an archangel.

"By stretching, we liberate our tensions, beneath which are hidden—more profoundly—Life, Love, and Joy, essential qualities of the human entity."

IDRIS LAHORE

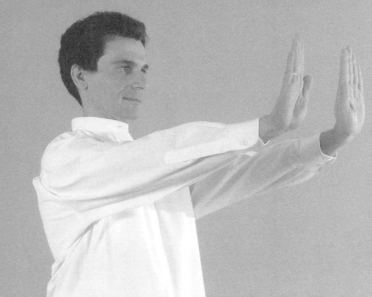

ARKANA 5

MAZDANA
STRETCHING OF THE JOY OF LIFE

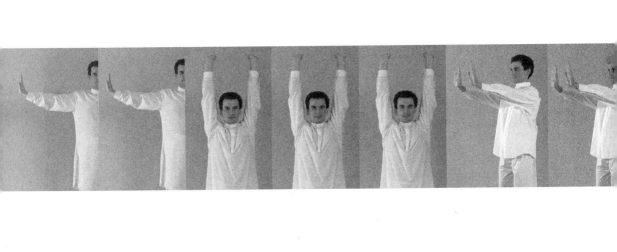

STRETCHING OF THE JOY OF LIFE

*This Arkana acts principally upon the skin, kidneys, and bladder.
It has a detoxifying action.*

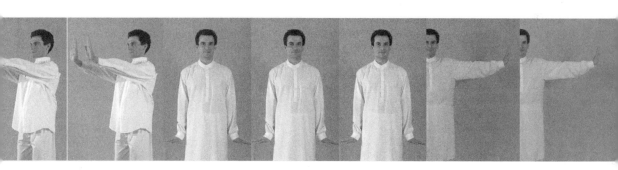

Passing from tension to relaxation induces, practically instantaneously,
a state of well-being.

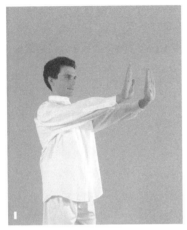 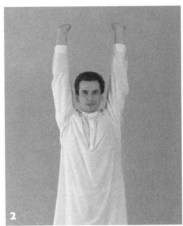 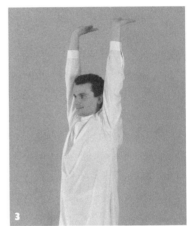

Begin the exercise in the fundamental position.

1) Lift your arms in front of you and stretch them, the palms of your hands facing forward.

2–3) Raise your arms and stretch them in the same way, your palms facing toward the sky.

In our muscular tensions are hidden the three fundamental negative emotions, inscribed in every one of us at birth. These three "poisons" are sadness, anger, and fear.

Relaxing our tensions permits us to liberate these negative layers, beneath which are hidden—more profoundly—life, love, and joy, true and essential qualities of mankind. Energy and joy are present beneath all of our tensions. Through work on our body, for example relaxation exercises (see pages 113–116), breathing exercises, or stretching exercises, we can gradually dissolve these tensions.

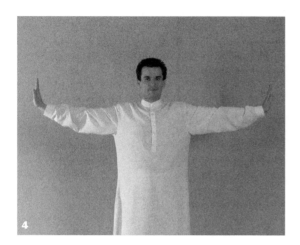 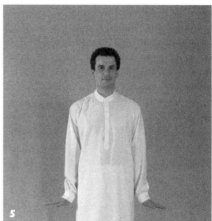

4) Now hold your arms out horizontally, your palms turned to the sides, and stretch once more.

5) Finally, hold your arms along the length of your body and stretch them a fourth time, your palms facing the ground.

Stretching is tension followed by relaxation. The tension created when we stretch has a homeopathic effect: we live with our tensions, most of the time without knowing it; when we do the stretching exercises, we create slightly more tension, and then the transition from tension to relaxation has a practically instantaneous effect of well-being.

"When we become conscious of our body, this can lead us to the realization that we are, as it were, a hieroglyph of the cosmos."

ENNEA TESS GRIFFITH

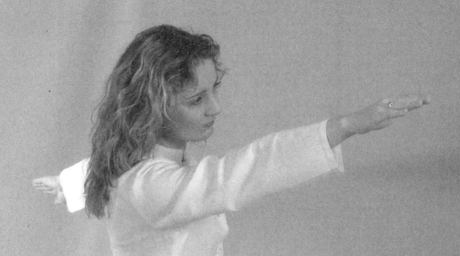

ARKANA 6

AHURA
SPARKS OF FIRE

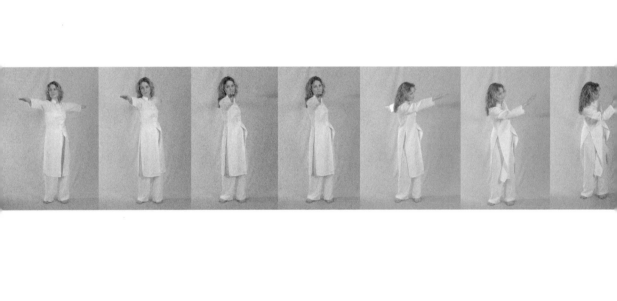

SPARKS OF FIRE

This Arkana acts principally upon the digestive and immune systems.
It also acts upon the back and neck and harmonizes the psyche.

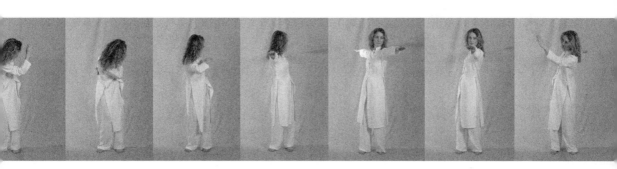

"Through the gateway of the senses
I may lead into my inmost soul
The word of worlds who speaks:
Fill thy spirit's depths
With my world expanse
To find hereafter me in thee."

—RUDOLF STEINER, "Calendar of the Soul"

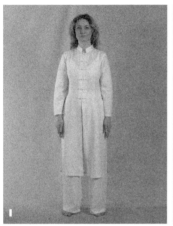
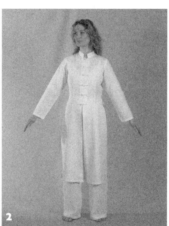
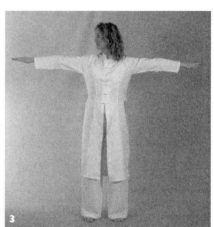

1) Begin in the fundamental position.

2-3) Raise your arms horizontally. Fix your gaze upon your right hand.

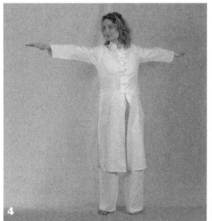
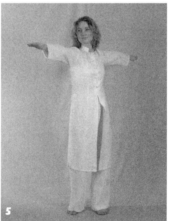
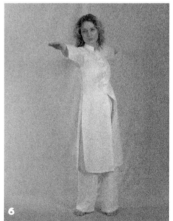

4–6) Rotate your torso to the left. Your arms follow the rotation, but remaining horizontal, in line with your shoulders. Your gaze remains fixed on your right hand.

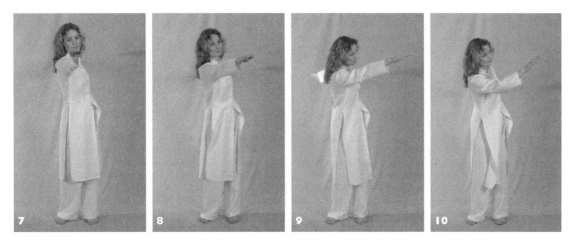

7–10) When your right arm is facing forward, start gradually bending your arms, at the same time lightly bending your knees.

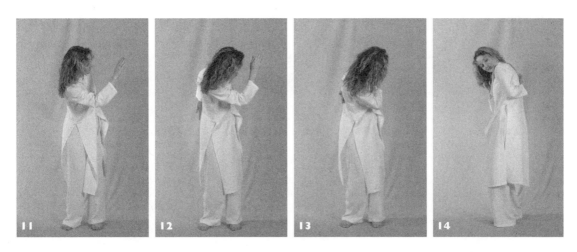

11–14) The movement of your torso carries along your hips, which rotate slightly to the left, until your right hand is placed on your left shoulder, and the back of your left hand—with a circular motion—on your right shoulder blade.

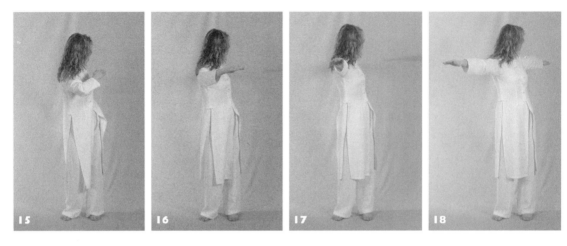

15–17) Gradually straighten your right arm forward and left arm backward—arriving at the sagittal plane—while straightening your head and torso. Your gaze now turns and rests upon your left hand.

18) Start rotating your torso in the opposite direction.

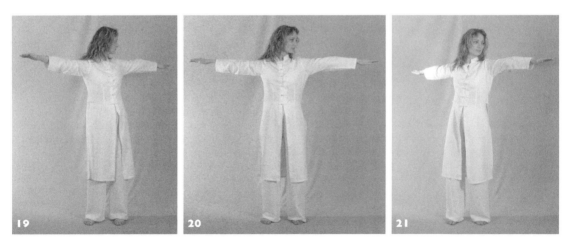

19–21) Continue the rotation, passing through the horizontal position...

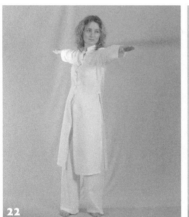
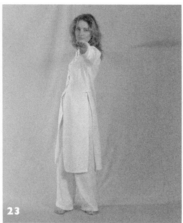
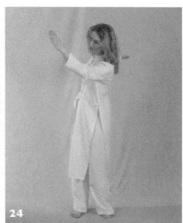

22) Continue the movement of rotation further, your gaze remaining upon your left hand.

23) You once again pass through the sagittal plane, your arms stretched out.

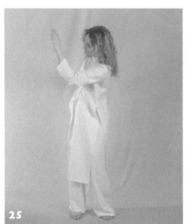
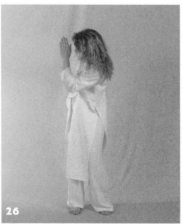
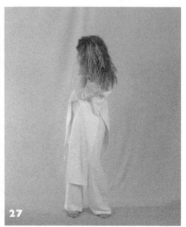

24–27) Continue the movement, bending your arms until your left hand rests upon your right shoulder and the back of your right hand, after tracing a circular motion, upon your left shoulder blade.

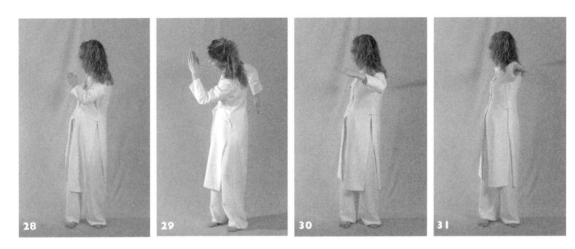

28–31) Gradually straighten your left arm forward and right arm backward—arriving at the sagittal plane—while straightening your head and torso. Your gaze now turns and rests upon your right hand.

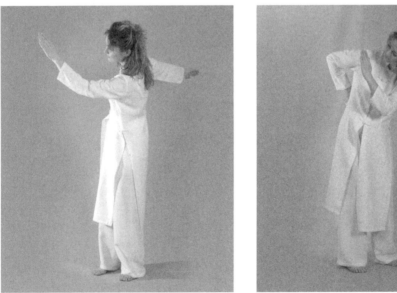

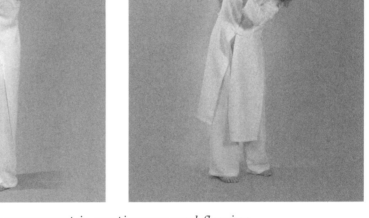

The movement is continuous and flowing.
Your arms trace circular movements in space.

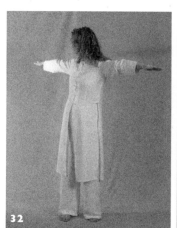
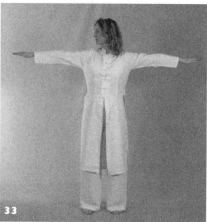
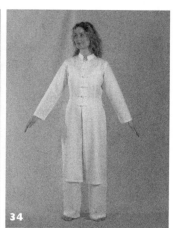

32–33) Start rotating your torso in the other direction. You pass again through the horizontal position...

Repeat this complete cycle (starting on page 94) five times.

34) When you have returned to the horizontal position for the last time, turn your head and look straight in front of you, then lower your arms along the length of your body.

When the movements begin to degenerate in our body, they harden, they rigidify in us. When the inner movement of our emotions and thoughts is no longer harmonious, this movement is also blocked, and hardens in the physical body.

The movements of Samadeva Gestural Euphony, and particularly the seven major Arkanas, archetypes of therapeutic, curative movements, slow the degeneration of the movements of the body, emotions, and thoughts, bringing them a new, reharmonizing, regenerative energy.

"Rumi fell into ecstasy, and he felt his own soul as it, too, began to whirl. He who had never danced before, who had never practiced the Sama, began whirling in the goldsmith's shop. For the first time, he recognized his own soul, which rose from his body, lifting him up toward the heavens."

IDRIS LAHORE, "Rumi and the Soul of the Goddess Samadeva"

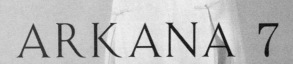

ARKANA 7

SAMA
DANCE OF THE PLANETS

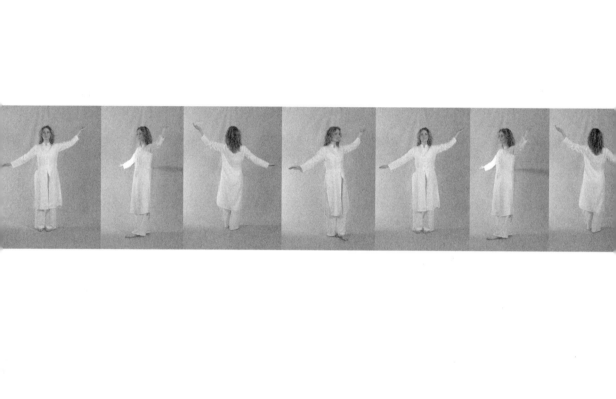

DANCE OF THE PLANETS

This Arkana principally reharmonizes the nervous and endocrine systems.
It harmonizes the psyche and brings physical well-being,
emotional purification, and intellectual clarity.

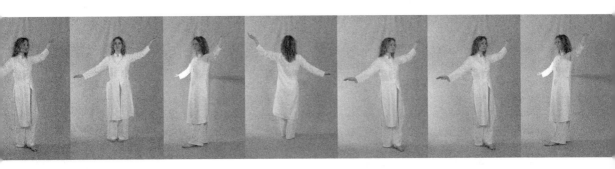

Sama, the whirling movement or whirling dance, is known especially thanks to the whirling dervishes of Konya. The *Sama* was taught to them by Rumi, the Master who was founder of their brotherhood. Through the *Sama,* we enter into resonance with the primordial movement of all things that are in movement, from the planets to the atoms. *Sama* is an exercise that gives us greater energy and intensity, wholeness, and a new joy of living. The *Sama* is said to fortify the body, purify the heart, and clarify the thoughts.

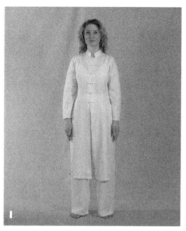
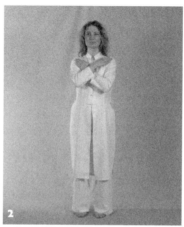
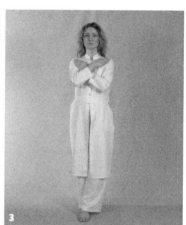

1) Relax for a few moments in the fundamental position.

2) Cross your arms over your chest. Your feet are close together.

3) Place your weight on your right foot, then raise your left foot and place it in front of your right foot, but slightly to the right of it, so that they are parallel. Your right foot is well-anchored in the ground.

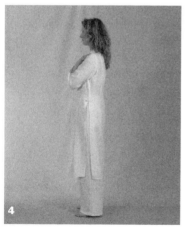
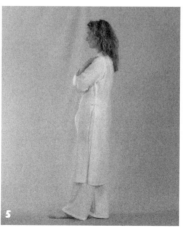
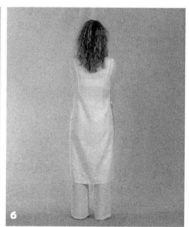

4) Your left foot gives the impetus for a quarter-turn to the right, while your right foot remains perfectly flat on the ground. Your right foot simply glides along while you are turning, it is never raised. Your body turns around the axis of your right foot.

5–6) Continue turning in this way, your right foot remaining flat on the ground and your left foot giving the impetus for quarter-turns to the right.

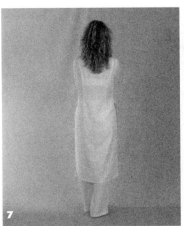 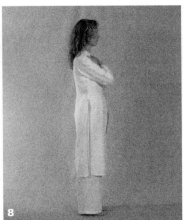 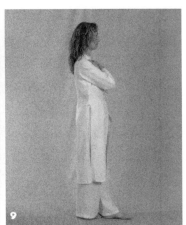

7–10) Continue turning to the right.

You may gradually accelerate the movement, replacing the quarter-turns with half-turns.

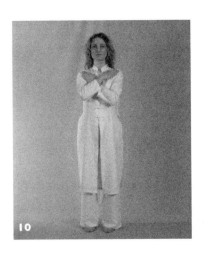

The *Sama* is to be learned in several stages, and it is essential to follow the progression from one stage to the next. The most important thing is to maintain your balance and for your right foot to remain in good contact with the ground. Breathe calmly and try to be inwardly peaceful. Learn at first to turn very slowly and consciously, in slow motion.

Note: You will need a little space in order to practice the *Sama*; make sure there are no objects or furniture in the way. At first it is best to practice on a smooth floor and to wear a pair of slippers or ballet shoes. Make sure that you are not interrupted at any moment while you are doing the exercise.

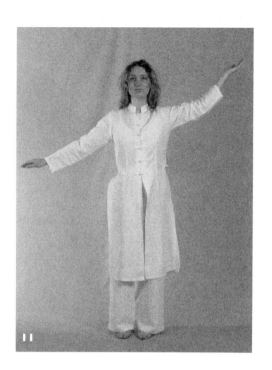
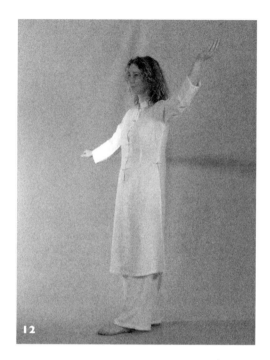

11–14) When you are comfortable doing the half-turns, spread out your arms, your left palm toward the sky and your right palm toward the earth. Turn at your own speed; you may accelerate until you find the rhythm you feel comfortable with, at which the motion is flowing. Raise your left foot from the ground and give the impulse for the rotation. It is important to first place your left foot on the ground and only turn afterwards. First pass your left foot over your right foot, place it on the ground, and turn; pass your left foot again over your right foot, place it on the ground, and turn… The faster you raise your left foot from the ground, the more the half-turns become flowing, complete turns.

Note: If, at the outset, you start feeling dizzy or nauseous, take a break. With practice, these sensations will disappear. If they do not disappear, you either have a psychosomatic problem or a physiological illness that ought to be addressed.

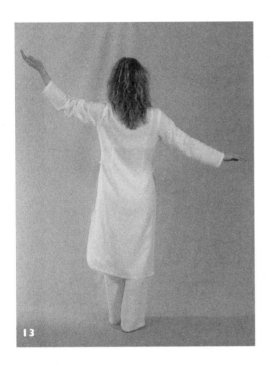
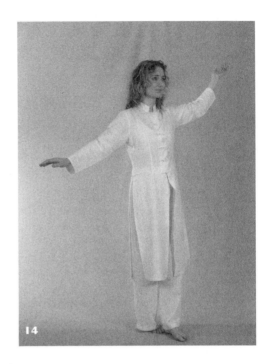

The beneficial effects of practicing the *Sama* include: improvement of one's general state, with a specific action upon visible problems; aid for healing and recovery; psychosomatic equilibrium; emotional liberation; improvement of sensory functioning; improvement of sexuality; disappearance of states of fear and distress; relativization of situations, which become less dramatic; alleviation of interpersonal difficulties; discovery of solutions; inner feeling of freedom; enhancement of creativity; positive transformation of dreams; and development of intuition and other extrasensory faculties.

The *Sama* is one of the most direct methods for purifying us of our negative emotions and rigid thought schemas. For those capable of practicing it, the Sama is worth all the therapies in the world. For the dervishes, *Sama* means to leave one's problems behind, elevating oneself toward their resolution.

RUMI AND THE SOUL OF THE GODDESS SAMADEVA

In his time, Rumi was considered to be the greatest poet, philosopher, and scholar of the Persian language; but up until then, his religious Puritanism had prevented him from becoming interested in the apparently more super-ficial manifestations of art, like music, dance, and song. One day he was walking through the streets of Konya when he saw a man dancing the Sama, the whirling dance of the dervishes. It was Shamz of Tabriz, who was to become his Master. Watching Shamz turn and practice his dancing exercises, Rumi fell into a state of ecstasy. He then had the following extraordinary vision: while Shamz was turning, Rumi saw a dancer step out of his body and rise toward the heavens, and he knew that this was the soul of Shamz.

From this moment dates Rumi's conversion to the whirling dance of the dervishes, which he was later to make the very heart of his teaching. Rumi's state of ecstasy lasted so long that by the time it had ended, Shamz had already disappeared. Distraught, Rumi went out in search of him. He walked the alleyways of the souk, one after the other, and passing by a goldsmith's shop, heard the crystalline patter of a tiny hammer tap-ping on gilded metal. He entered the shop and perceived, beside the goldsmith, a young girl hammering an object she was holding in her hands.

Coming closer, Rumi saw that she was sculpting a dancer, the perfect replica of the dancer he had recognized earlier as the soul of Shamz of Tabriz. Once again, Rumi fell into ecstasy and felt his own soul as it, too, began to whirl. He who had never danced before, who had never practiced the Sama, began whirling in the goldsmith's shop. For the first time, he recognized his own soul, which, like the soul of Shamz, rose from his body, lifting him up toward the heavens. After the state of ecstasy had come to an end, Rumi remained for a time with the goldsmith and his daughter. He learned that she was sculpting the dancer Samadeva, one of the Hindu goddesses of the dance

According to the legend of Samadeva, the human soul is naturally beautiful and joyous, but imprisoned, as it were, in the physical body with all its limitations and illnesses, and prisoner also of many negative and conflictual emotions. The Samadeva dances and exercises liberate this soul. Man's thoughts become clear, his emotions positive, and his body young and healthy once again.

Such is the tale of the dancer Samadeva, recognized as the goddess of the dance by the wandering dervishes, the Malamati dervishes of South India, the brotherhood to which Shamz of Tabriz belonged. The mystical dancers say that by turning, by practicing these dances, the dancer is united with the soul of the dance, with the goddess of the dance, with Samadeva.

COMPLEMENTARY
ARKANA

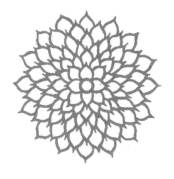

SAPRANA
RELAXATION

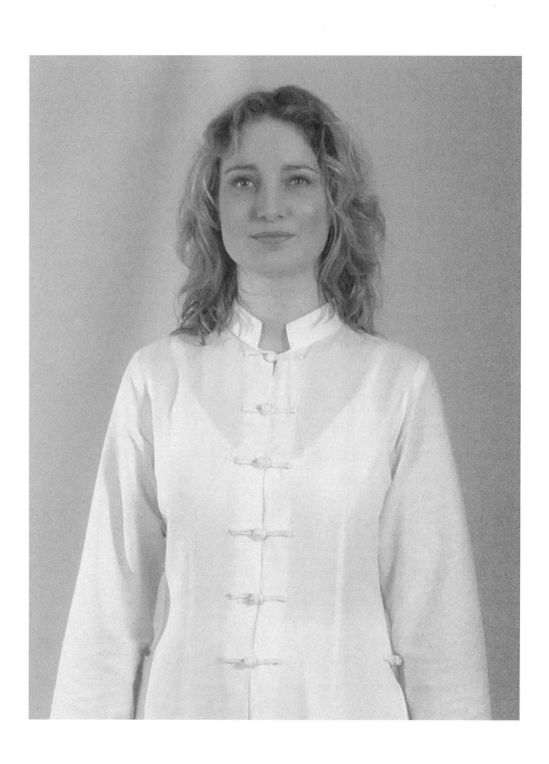

SAPRANA: RELAXATION

For any kind of activity, whether physical, intellectual, or emotional, you need energy. In order to have a sufficient amount of energy, it makes sense to avoid dispersing it uselessly, to avoid wasting it, and this is especially true for your muscular tensions. Learn to relax by practicing simple exercises, such as the following seated or lying down relaxations.

Seated relaxation

Sit down comfortably in a chair that allows you to adopt and maintain a vertical position. Place your hands flat on your knees. You may rest your lower back on the back of the chair, but make sure your vertebral column is straight, without forcing and without tension. Your head should be aligned with your vertebral column and your eyes should remain open; start by trying to relax the tensions in your face, neck, and body.

To free the tensions in your eyes, try to perceive your eyes intensively, as if you were entering into them. Be present to your eyes, sense them, really feel them. Now you can relax them and relax your eye muscles as well. Keep your eyes open, but don't stare at any particular object.

To free your facial tensions, become aware of your face as a whole, and of your mouth. One by one, relax each part of your face that you can think of. Let each part of your face relax.

To relax the tensions in your neck, shoulders, and hands, first feel your neck muscles, then relax them. Feel your right shoulder, then relax it; do the same for your left shoulder, and then with your right and left hands. Feel each muscle, then relax it.

Now place your awareness in the muscles from your chest to your diaphragm, and relax them.

Relax your abdominal muscles and notice how your breathing is becoming deeper and calmer. You are gradually becoming calmer. Move on to your right leg, from your thigh down to your foot, and then to your left leg.

Do all of this very slowly so that you are able to really feel each part of your body. Feel as your whole body is becoming relaxed, feel the weight of your relaxed body. You are present to your body, you are conscious of your body.

When you repeat the exercise a second time, try to enter even more profoundly into each part of your body, down to your nervous system and blood circulation. You will notice a sensation of heat or tingling in certain parts of your body.

To come out of the exercise, breathe deeply once or twice.

Note: This exercise may be practiced daily. Twenty to thirty sessions are necessary in order to practice it correctly. When you have acquired the habit of doing the exercise, you can reduce its length without losing any of its benefits.

Lying down relaxation

Lie down on your back, your legs straight; rest your head on a small pillow so that your neck is in line with your vertebral column. Your arms are resting along the sides of your body, the palms of your hands toward the ground.

Start by relaxing your face: relax your forehead, then your eyelids and cheek muscles, then move on to your jaws and the muscles of your mouth, which may open slightly, and relax your tongue. Your whole face is relaxed. Relax the muscles of your neck.

Now concentrate on your right arm. Relax your right shoulder, then relax the muscles of your upper arm, forearm, hand, and fingers. Your entire right arm is now relaxed.

Move on to your left arm. Relax your left shoulder, then relax the muscles of your upper arm, forearm, hand, and fingers. Both your arms are lying on the ground, relaxed.

Now concentrate on your back, on its points of contact with the ground. Relax the muscles along the length of your vertebral column.

Relax the muscles of your chest, stomach, and lower abdomen. Your breathing becomes calm, slow, and deep.

Concentrate on your right leg, and relax the muscles of your buttocks, thigh, calf, and foot.

Then concentrate on your left leg, and relax the muscles of your buttocks, thigh, calf, and foot.

At present your entire body is relaxed and resting calmly on the ground. You may be filled with a feeling of calm, peace, and harmony, a feeling that can remain with you after the relaxation is over.

You may continue the exercise until you gradually fall asleep. You may also choose to come out of the exercise by breathing deeply once or twice. After breathing deeply, move your fingers and toes and stretch yourself pleasantly, like after a good night's sleep, and your muscles are once again ready for activity.

Open your eyes to return with pleasure to the reality that surrounds you. You are regenerated and full of vitality.

If you practice this relaxation exercise regularly, you will save a great quantity of conscious energy.

COMPLEMENTARY ARKANA

DYANA MEDITATION

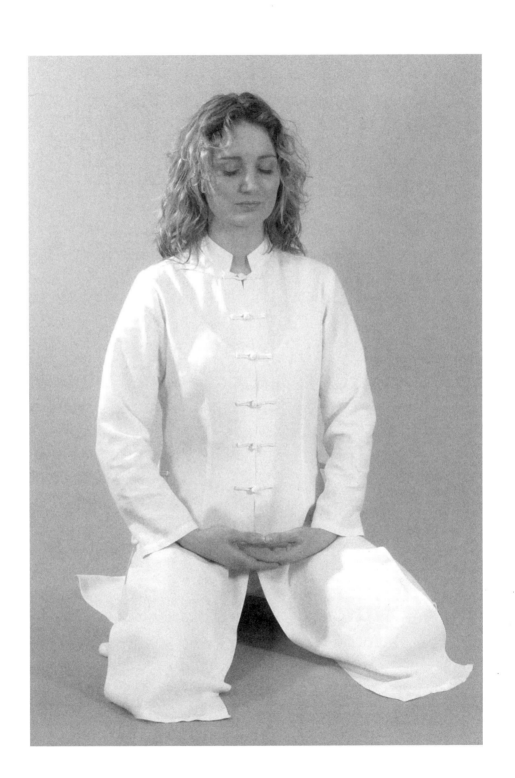

THE POSTURE
OF MEDITATION

Sit down onto your legs and feet, your knees spread and in line with your hips. Tilt your pelvis forward to arch your lower back slightly in order to ensure that your vertebral column is straight, but without tensing your muscles. In order to find this position, you may tilt forward and backward, gradually reducing the movement until you are seated comfortably. Your neck is straight, slightly extended, and your chin is slightly tucked in. Close your eyes. Relax your face and the muscles of your eyes and forehead. Unclench your jaws and lips, as if you were smiling inwardly. Place one hand in the other, and relax your arms and shoulders. Find the right level of tension in your body, which should be minimal, without any strain; you should be balanced and vertical, but not rigid. The posture is at once strong and supple, upright and alive. It is by no means slack, but neither is it forced.

Breathe from your lower abdomen; center yourself on the exhale, which should be slow and deep, but without forcing. The inhale comes naturally and deeply. The exhale should be twice as long as the inhale, with a retention of two seconds between inhale and exhale.

The meditation consists in being conscious of your breathing while remaining as immobile as possible. When thoughts or emotions come during the meditation, this is not a problem; simply let them pass, like clouds in the sky, without following them, and return to your breathing.

Note: Meditation is practiced for twenty minutes, one to three times daily.

When you have finished your sitting, turn your head gently to the left and right, rub your hands together, tilt your body to the left and right, forward and backward, then bend forward, free your legs, move your joints a little, and finally stand up, walking in place for a few moments.

In order to be more conscious of your breathing during the meditation:

You can let the air pass gently through your larynx, making a continuous, soft, blowing sound during the exhale. Your breathing then becomes slower and deeper, and if you concentrate well on the air passing through your larynx and the quiet sound it makes, your concentration will improve. You can practice this more loudly when you first start meditating and more discreetly later on.

In order to improve your concentration:

You may focus your attention on your lower abdomen, in the region of the vital center or *hara*. You can feel how the hara, located a few centimeters below the navel, hardens during the exhale. This also helps to improve concentration. If you relax your shoulders at the same time, at the beginning of the exhale, and allow yourself to glide downward as if you were trying to sit more comfortably, you will be in the correct position. Relax your shoulders, lower yourself, and sit down; at the same time, extend your neck slightly, tuck in your chin, and raise the top of your head toward the sky. Then it is as if, in exhaling, your breath were to ascend from deep within your lower abdomen, with the result that your abdomen is drawn inward, tensing slightly. It is important to avoid forcing; exhale as completely as possible, but without forcing, and then the inhale comes naturally, also without forcing.

The direct experience of consciousness of self

Man's normal state is to have thoughts. Usually he takes himself to be his thoughts, he mistakes himself for them. He is his thoughts, he is not the one who is thinking. As long as he remains in this state, it is impossible for him to attain anything higher. He has to part from the realm of the thoughts constantly going around in circles inside his head and attain to the thinker himself, at a distance from his thoughts. The goal of meditation is to arrive at this direct experience of consciousness of self. The I becomes conscious of itself, it sees itself at a distance from its thoughts. By transcending the level of ordinary, mechanical thoughts, he raises himself to the level of consciousness.

We know that it is impossible to stop the constant flow of thoughts and enter directly into consciousness, since the thoughts act as a barrier between oneself and one's spirit. So it is necessary to go through them, as it were, to "transcend" them, without suppressing them in the process. This is possible through the techniques of meditation.

During meditation, it is important to direct your inner activity toward something other than the desires of your ego. Your mind must become innerly receptive, and it must also stop losing itself in all the sensations coming to you from the external world. Stop the internal chatter and start listening... If thoughts come all the same, this is not important, provided you do not follow them. When you have the habit of doing this, you will enter into higher levels of consciousness naturally. But this cannot be forced, it happens ... simply by concentrating on your breathing.

ARKANA
OF SEXUALITY

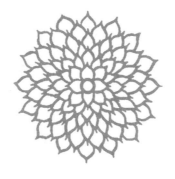

OM SAMADEVA

THE ARKANA OF SEXUALITY

The Arkana of sexuality is of Taoist origin. The Chinese sages considered it to be the exercise of longevity par excellence—they taught that each month of regular practice prolongs the practitioner's life by one year. It permits To, the universal energy, to be attracted into the sexual center, where To unites with Qi, the vital energy of man. The exercise was to be necessarily accompanied by a breathing exercise that was only revealed to initiates, in addition to a vocal exercise consisting in the repetition of certain sacred syllables.

The breathing exercise, practiced exclusively by the masters, consisted in extracting the most subtle substance from the air inhaled, the prana of To, into Latifa Lalana, through the use of sacred syllables made to resonate in the larynx. The prana of To was subsequently sent along the length of the vertebral column toward the second chakra, the sexual center, where upon contacting Qi, the sexual energy, it underwent an alchemical process of transformation before being directed toward the ninth chakra, Binduvisarga, at the back of the head.

According to the Taoist tradition, this resulted in the birth of a second, subtle and energetic body which was to gradually replace the physical body. This second body, as it was not of a terrestrial and material nature, was held to be immortal. These techniques were later used by most of the great spiritual currents of the East and Middle East. We can also find traces of them in the Hindu Vedanta, the repetitions of the Buddhist Nembutsu, the Prayer of the Heart of Orthodox Christian monks, and the Sufi Dikhr.

The Masters of Wisdom, the Sarmans, through the intermediary of the Malamati dervishes who travelled from India to Iran via Pakistan and Afghanistan, transmitted these techniques to the Muslim Sufis, and particularly to the Kwajaghan brotherhood, to which Bahauddin Naqshband of Bokhara belonged. Bahauddin was the founder of the tarika of Naqshbandi Sufis, who have had a considerable influence upon all Middle Eastern civilizations.

Each of these currents sensibly modified the original technique of the Taoist masters, adapting it not only to initiates but to all the men and women who so desired and were capable of making the effort of practicing it. In this book we present it in a form that is adapted to the men and women of today.

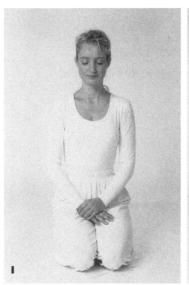 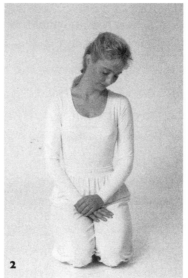 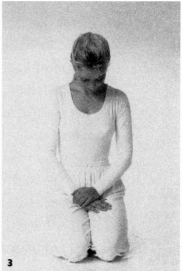

1) Sit down on your knees, your legs tucked under your body. Hold your right wrist in your left hand. Your head is held straight, in line with your vertebral column.

2) Lower your head, tilting your left cheek toward your left shoulder while pronouncing the syllable OM.

When it is practiced regularly but not excessively, this special exercise brings about a harmonization of the physical, emotional, and intellectual functions connected to sexuality. Through a gentle action upon the chakra *Latifa Lalana* and the chakra *Binduvisarga*, the sexual center is restored to a state of equilibrium. This results in either a calming or stimulation of the sexual functions, according to what is needed.

In addition to the seven chakras we have studied, there exist many others distributed throughout the human organism. We mentioned the eighth chakra, Latifa Lalana, which secretes the "elixir of long life" (see page 28). On the back of the head, the ninth chakra, Binduvisarga, can be found. Like Latifa Lalana, it is very mysterious, since it is associated with the production of the

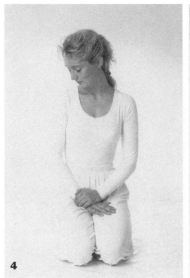
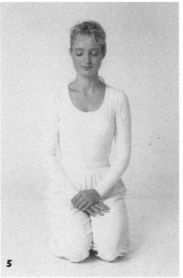
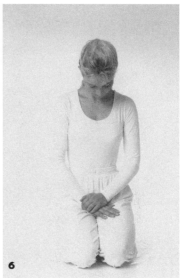

3–4) Move your head in a semicircular motion toward your right shoulder while pronouncing the syllables SAMA.

5) Straighten your head into the vertical position while pronouncing the syllable DE.

6) Lower your head downward, toward your heart, pronouncing the syllable VA.

male semen (*bindu* means "drop of semen"). It is also called *somachakra*. Latifa Lalana and the chakra Binduvisarga have a close relationship with the second chakra, the sexual center (see pages 22–23) and the harmonious distribution of sexual energy, not only to the physical body, but also to the thoughts and emotions. Too much or too little energy in the second chakra causes most sexual problems, such as impotence, frigidity, and sterility.

An energetic disequilibrium in Latifa Lalana leads to such forms of emotional disharmony as indifference and jealousy. An energetic disequilibrium in the chakra Binduvisarga causes problems in thoughts and behaviors connected to sexuality, such as fixed ideas, obsessions, exhibitionism, and so on.

COMMENTARY

ON SAMADEVA GESTURAL EUPHONY

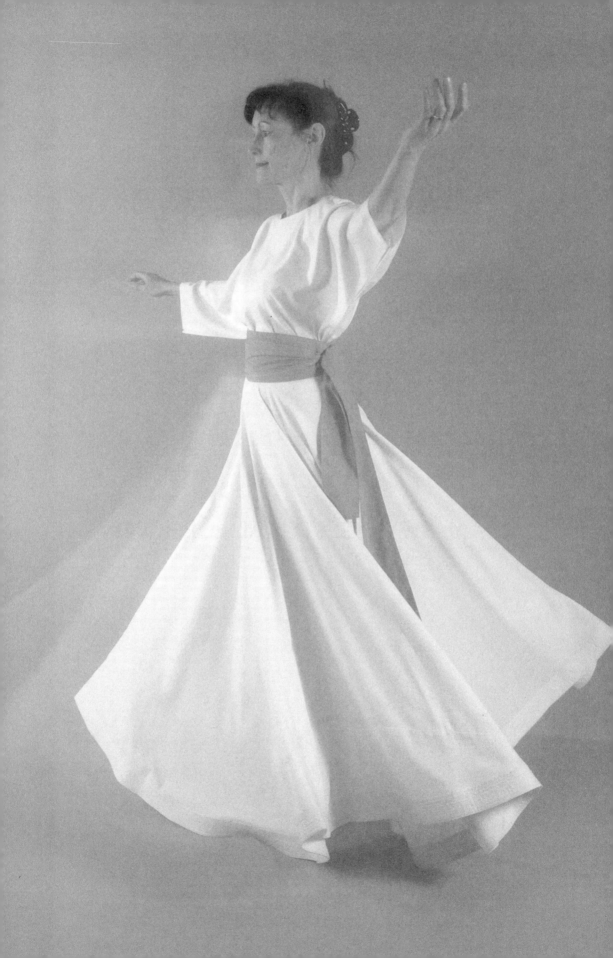

THE HEART OF
SAMADEVA GESTURAL EUPHONY:
THE "MODEL SESSION"

The harmonizing, structuring, and therapeutic effects observed during the regular practice of the seven major Arkanas are even more remarkable when they are practiced in the context of a "model session."

The "model session," heart of Samadeva Gestural Euphony

The heart of Samadeva Gestural Euphony, the model session is designed to meet the most vital needs of men and women today.

The regular practice of the seven major Arkanas in the context of a model session not only augments their positive physical, psychological, and energetic effects, but also permits us to enter into a deeper and more intense state of listening, of listening to ourselves; in this way we enter into contact with our own being and inner wisdom, which we most of the time stifle, becoming identified with our emotions, mechanical thoughts, and actions, or escaping into frenzied activity and all kinds of superficial pursuits.

The nine phases of the model session

A model session, which lasts an hour and fifteen minutes, has nine phases:

- In order to return to an inner state of calm, the session begins with five minutes of immobility, during which the participant is centered on his or her breathing.

- Exercises to relax the neck and an energetic exercise for the hands.

- Stretching exercises accompanied by specific breathing.

- Dynamic exercises which train especially a simultaneous attention to rhythm, coordination, and the sense of space.

- The major Arkanas.

- Meditative Movements (slow movements tracing the letters of the alphabet in space).

- Five minutes seated silently, centered again on the breathing (see pages 119–122).

- An Arkana of relaxation (see pages 113–116).

- A space of possible exchange between the participants, lasting around ten minutes, respecting each person and his or her differences, called the "circle of respect."

When we practice the seven major Arkanas regularly in the context of a model session, we very soon experience their harmonizing, structuring, and therapeutic effects.

INDICATIONS AND COUNTERINDICATIONS

Idris Lahore

Samadeva Gestural Euphony combines many different techniques whose importance is evident for one's therapeutic arsenal in both the physical and psychological domains. The diversity of the exercises permits an extremely flexible and individual adaptation according to the possible indications and counterindications.

In each case, the indications and counterindications are to be specified so that the exercises may be used preventatively, curatively, and palliatively according to the individuality of each participant and the specific features of his illness.

indications   Indications include the following:

- Osteo-articulatory pathologies (lumbar pain, dorsalgia, rheumatism), taking into account possible precautions and counterindications.

- Cardiovascular pathologies (venous and arterial problems, rhythmic problems, high blood-pressure).

- Nervous pathologies and behavioral disorders, such as nervousness, spasmophilia, anxiety, fear, depression, lack of concentration, and so on.

- ENT and respiratory pathologies: various problems with a tendency to become chronic (rhinitis, allergies, asthma, and so on).

- Gynecological and obstetric pathologies, especially hormonal dysfunctions. Certain exercises may also be used as an aid for the preparation of childbirth.

- Digestive pathologies, especially all problems of a psychosomatic nature, from ulcers to gastritis, enterocolitis, colopathy, and so on.

- More serious pathologies (oncology and immunal problems); in such cases, Samadeva Gestural Euphony is used as a secondary or adjunct treatment.

Samadeva Gestural Euphony, consisting of a number of highly effective techniques from a psychosomatic point of view, has in spite of this certain counterindications, specifically epilepsy, Parkinson's disease, Ménière's syndrome, certain cardiac, circulatory, rheumatic, and infectious pathologies, and certain psychiatric pathologies. In each of these cases, the prior authorization of the attending physician is necessary. Certain exercises may be practiced, while others must be absolutely avoided.

Temporary counterindications are the following: advanced pregnancy, a recent heart attack, and surgery within the past six months.

counterindications

PHENOMENOLOGY

Idris Lahore

A range of phenomena may occur during the practice of Samadeva Gestural Euphony, for example:

- An emotional-kinetic liberation, in the form of psycho-motor expressions such as laughing or crying, or a disinhibition involving exuberant movements, particularly in the case of timid persons. These manifestations become less pronounced as practice continues, to be replaced by calmer and more harmonious expressions.

- Anesthesia (analgesia), in which certain parts of the body are no longer sensitive to pain, and sustained or even violent effort is experienced positively as increasing the sensation of pleasure or well-being (compare endorphins).

- A gaze turned inward, typical of phenomena of religious, ritual, or artistic ecstasy.

- Artistic exhibitionism as an epiphenomenon typical of the choreographic expression of existential or emotional situations.

- Impression of distortion of time, in the sense of reduction—the participant thinks a few minutes have passed, whereas the exercises have lasted an hour-and-a-half.

- Impression of distortion of space, in the sense of widening, with a transformation of the perception of the body schema (impression that the body is larger, smaller, or lighter, and so on).

- Nonhypnotic regression of memory, with the surfacing of childhood memories which, when positive, augment the sense of well-being and, when negative, are experienced as the liberation and elimination of a toxic element.

- Daydreaming accompanied by a calming and harmonizing effect, often described as "wonderful."

- Perception of colors and light, or visualization of oneself as in the experiences of deep relaxation in autogenic training or Zen meditation.

OPTIMIZE YOUR HEALTH

Idris Lahore

In order to stay physically fit, we recommend exercising regularly. Small, daily efforts are preferable to occasional extreme efforts.

Our physical exercises can be practiced by young and vigorous individuals, but also by older people with less strength; they can always be adapted to the condition of the person practicing them.

In your everyday life, try to maintain a good posture at all times, whether you are standing up, sitting, walking, or lying down. Make an effort to relax as often as possible; concentrate often on relaxing your face, back, cheeks, and jaws. Make it a principle for your face to be relaxed and not tense; likewise, remember often to relax your hands, fingers, and palms. Relax often, very often. By relaxing in this way, you will save a great deal of energy. In addition, relaxation improves blood circulation throughout your whole body.

think about relaxing your tensions as often as possible

A good night's sleep regenerates our entire psychological and physiological organism. At the same time, it allows our unconscious to pass on various messages, in the form of dreams, to our conscious I. We should be attentive to these messages, since they can sometimes offer valuable guidance for our everyday lives. Dreams occur during cer-

be attentive to the quality of your sleep

tain sleep phases; they regulate and purify our conscious life, but for those who meditate, it is not necessary to interpret them, even if they have great importance as a phenomenon of observation.

Science has shown us that even during sleep, our brain is not entirely at rest, but that the more our brain activity slows down, the more we tend to fall asleep—unless we hold our neck straight, in line with our vertebral column, when we are seated in meditation. Nonetheless, as soon as our head and neck start tilting downward, we run the risk of falling asleep, even during meditation.

A good night's sleep is necessary for good physical and psychological health. Unfortunately, more and more people today suffer from insomnia; like stress, it is one of the plagues of our modern civilization. We know that without a good regenerative sleep, our entire nervous system is unable to function properly, and when our nervous system is unbalanced, we are unable to live in peace.

The main factors responsible for disturbing our sleep are nervous and psychological tensions caused by worries, excessive consumption of tea and coffee, late-night meals, lack of physical exercise, noise and commotion, intellectual overload, television, radio, listening to music before going to bed, sexual imbalance (either too much or too little), incorrect and superficial breathing, and a poor-quality mattress (often too soft).

factors that disturb our sleep

We can improve our sleep by not eating after seven o'clock P.M. and drinking herbal teas made from plants with a mildly calming effect, such as valerian, passionflower, orange flower, or lime blossom. We can also take up the habit of light physical exercise, such as the evening walk, work in the garden, or calm housekeeping work, and practice breathing exercises like deep, abdominal respiration, or use a relaxation method before going to sleep.

how to improve our sleep

The quality of our diet is also important; most people in our society are overfed, so for those who wish to improve or maintain their health, it is necessary to eat less. Eating too much puts unnecessary strain on our stomach, intestines, and liver, all of which need extra energy for digestion. As a result, this energy is not available for the life of the spirit. The first important principle is to eat moderately, and the second is to chew your food well, thanks to which it will be more easily digested. The third principle is to refrain from taking your meals after seven o'clock in the evening. The fourth principle is to choose your food well; it is best if your diet consists primarily of organically- or biodynamically-grown grains and vegetables, regional fruits, yogurt, and organic cold-pressed vegetable oils. Avoid sweets made from white sugar, chocolate, canned foods, and industrially-produced foods. Dairy products and eggs should be consumed in moderation. As far as consumption of meat is concerned, it is better to abstain if you are able to do so. The fifth principle is to avoid, as much as possible, chemical medications, coffee, cigarettes, alcohol, and other drugs.

the quality of our diet

Food should be considered above all as a means to maintain the cells, tissues, and organs of the body in a healthy state of functioning. You should try to eliminate any form of psychological dependency on certain foods and drinks (wine, beer, chocolate, pastries, and so on); then your body itself will give you signs concerning the diet that is adapted to your own individual needs.

what to avoid

It is necessary to understand that man's real energy does not come from the food he eats, but from the spirit. Eating a sufficient amount of food is important, provided you adhere to the above-mentioned principles. Nonetheless, each person is different and needs to conscientiously examine these principles for himself in order to apply them in the best possible way.

eat lightly

It is advisable to drink two to three liters of fluids daily, in the form of pure water, herbal or fruit teas, and fruit and vegetable juices.

drink in sufficient quantity

Fasting should not be practiced ascetically, but as a way to purify the body. One day a week is ideal. On this day, eat nothing and drink only liquids (pure water or herbal teas). For people with weaker constitutions and who tend to light-headedness, a day of fruit or fresh vegetable juice can replace a day of fasting. If you wish to fast for a longer period, you should consult your doctor.

fasting

We recommend that you wear, as much as possible, clothes made of natural, organic fabrics that are appropriate to each season. When it is cold, dress accordingly, paying particular attention to your neck; never go out into the cold directly after having washed your hair, and try to keep your feet warm at all times, avoiding cold drafts.

In conclusion, it should be mentioned that the fullness of life can only be experienced by someone who finds a balance between activity and rest, eating and drinking, hot and cold...

SCULPTING YOUR SOUL

Idris Lahore

always be at peace with
yourself and with other
people

Now some practical tips for sculpting your soul. Try
always to be at peace with yourself and with other
people. Do everything you can to be forgiving; this also
means trying to love other people, and acting in such a way
that they will love you. Be genuinely tolerant of other people and of yourself. Stop making a problem out of every situation; let things flow. Take life seriously, but don't take its
problems seriously—in any case, don't make tragedies out
of them.

learn to let go

> *One day, a prince who was fond of extravagant
> things summoned his counsellors.*
>
> *"Last night I dreamed of a ring," he told them,
> "that could make me happy when I was sad, but
> also a little sad when I was happy."*
>
> *And he told them to make him such a ring.*
>
> *Neither the counsellors, nor the ministers, nor
> the jewellers knew where to begin. So they sum-
> moned a dervish who was known for his wisdom.*
>
> *The dervish took a simple gold ring and
> engraved on it the words, "All things pass."*

("The Magic Ring," a dervish story)

Live and let live, try to make as few demands as possible of other people, leave them their freedom, and feel yourself free. The great philosopher Socrates said, "Those who make the fewest demands on other people are the most beloved of the gods." Try to be satisfied and happy about the smallest thing, and you will be all the happier when greater things happen to you. In addition, negative things will disturb you less and less.

make as few demands as possible of other people

be satisfied with the smallest thing

Cultivate a feeling of gratitude for everything you have, for everything that was passed on to you by your parents and by your ancestors, teachers, citizens of your country, and friends, without demanding or regretting whatever they have not given you.

cultivate a feeling of gratitude

When you look at other people, always see their positive qualities; see their faults, too, but don't remain attached to them. In the same way, cultivate your own positive qualities, your talents and gifts, and this will allow you to more easily forget all your faults and inadequacies.

always see the positive qualities in other people

If you observe faults in yourself, simply try to correct them, without having an inferiority complex or feeling guilty. If you are unable to do this, apply the method described above: develop your gifts, abilities, and talents. When we recommend that you cultivate your gifts, abilities, and talents, this means to be creative. Don't let yourself get bored, find something to do, even if you have to invent something, but don't remain idle.

develop your gifts, talents, and abilities

be creative

Tell yourself that the less you worry, the better you will live your life. If you have difficulties or problems, make the effort to examine them clearly or find someone who can help you to do so; then make a firm decision about how to deal with the problem, and don't let yourself deviate from it. If your problem does not have a solution, there is nothing else for you to do but accept it and live as best you can. In life, it is necessary to have the courage to change what you can change, and the strength to calmly and wisely accept what you cannot change.

the courage to change what you can change and the wisdom to accept what you cannot change

Cultivate your sense of humor; not mockery, sarcasm, or irony, but your sense of humor; begin with yourself, learn to laugh at yourself. But don't laugh at other people, laugh with them. If you feel like crying, even if you're a man, then cry; when you cry, you become a little more yourself.

cultivate your sense of humor

Try to be attentive to your breathing as often as possible, and to your way of walking, your words, and gestures. You will be astonished at how this attention, if practiced regularly, will give you the strength of inner calm, as well as a greater knowledge of yourself, other people, and the world.

be attentive

FROM CATHARSIS TO CONSCIOUSNESS

Ennea Tess Griffith

consciousness of the body: the port of entry for self-knowledge

The most crucial element when practicing Samadeva Gestural Euphony is for us to be conscious of our body, permitting us to enter into conscious relation with our psyche (our thoughts and emotions) and opening a path toward self-knowledge. This consciousness, developed by progressively refining our perception of our inner body, reharmonizes both our physical body and psyche, allowing us to rediscover new dimensions, a new vitality, and a new creativity in ourselves.

Rediscovering the Connection between Body and Spirit

Our work is carried out along two lines, in which a global approach to the body and psyche of man becomes apparent: firstly, methods of passive relaxation and active meditation, and secondly, dynamic movements and dances.

In order to gradually acquire a more refined consciousness of our body, one of the exercises' most essential aspects is their application, their adaptation to our everyday lives. The work done during a session can be concretely adapted to all of life's situations. The aim of the exercises thus goes beyond consciousness of the body alone, offering a valuable contribution to man's better integration into his material and interpersonal environment.

An important question can be raised: what is our position concerning psychological problems that may reveal themselves during such work?

We do not attempt to bring memories to the surface, nor to analyse the possible causes of blockages, but rather to help man as much as possible to reharmonize his body, to restore him to a state of health, connecting him to his psyche once again. This enables him to better experience and express the tensions that had, earlier, been suppressed. Thus Samadeva Gestural Euphony does not invite him to delve into his past, searching for the causes behind his physical tensions, but helps him instead to better deal with his present and future.

the body and its
connections to the psyche

Relaxation is important because it creates certain states that allow psychological maturation and clarification, further promoted by the stimulating and liberating effect of the dynamic exercises. These dynamic exercises are performed while remaining in contact with the environment—that is to say, with our eyes open—in contrast to the relaxation exercises. The individual is thus placed in a dynamic relationship with his body and environment, to which he is asked to adapt himself as well as possible.

Especially worthy of emphasis is the widening, the extension of the very idea of the body in Samadeva Gestural Euphony; the body is no longer considered to be a simple aggregation of material particles, a construction of mere flesh and bones. If we are, indeed, very much interested in the physical body, improving its joint flexibility and muscle extension (as in traditional gymnastics), we are also interested in the manifestation of rhythmic, respiratory, circulatory, and psychological phenomena. It becomes clear that the physical body can only move because vital forces are at work, permitting the organism to live and grow. We also perceive to an ever greater extent that our body is closely connected to our inner experiences, which are the basis of our sensations and feelings and give rise to our mental representations and thoughts. This is why we do not ignore the importance of the information received from our senses and bodily sensations; quite to the contrary, we make use of them in order to refine our consciousness of our body, emotions, and thoughts.

the phenomenon of catharsis

Let us try to better understand what takes place in certain psycho-corporal methods. Consider someone practicing a form of relaxation: stretched out on the floor, his eyes closed, partially hypnotized by the music or a monotonous voice calling forth images he cannot control. Man is placed here in a dream-like state of consciousness, image consciousness, the consciousness that was his in a distant past. This kind of relaxation thus invokes man's ancestral faculty of calling forth images from his psyche without the intervention of his conscious mental control. So we can understand why, during such relaxation sessions, a flood of images with no apparent relation to each other often enters the consciousness. We can also understand how these chaotic images affect the person's psyche; he is in a state in which he is at the mercy of the flood of images and representations originating in his unconscious, without the light of conscious thought to arrange or organize them.

Another aspect also becomes clear, namely the well-known phenomenon of catharsis, important in so many corporal therapies, during which an action upon a physical tension provokes an uncontrolled emotional release; the fact of touching a muscular blockage effectively provokes images connected to the origin of the tension. The "I" does not impose itself upon the perception-image-action sequence, it does not intentionally make an image of how it wants to act before the actual action takes place. If these images are not reflected upon by the light of conscious thought, the same phenomenon will occur that we find in animals: a kind of short-circuit between perception and action, a sensory perception which becomes a force compelling the animal to act immediately according to its momentary sympathy (attraction) or antipathy (aversion). Thus the uncontrolled gestures, crises, and tears.

from catharsis to consciousness

So we can foresee the danger posed by work that limits itself to bringing repressed feelings and buried impulses to the surface, soliciting an undeciphered flood of images from the unconscious. We run the risk of seeing the individual lose himself completely in the subjectivity of his own inner experiencings, the tangle of his ever-moving inner depths. In addition, the primary place accorded the unconscious can give the illusion of finding, in all of these inner movements, the real solution to our need for being and self-expression: don't we feel that we exist through the affective movements that agitate our soul? There is thus the danger of the individual bottling himself up, egoistically, in his own inner world, contenting himself with it alone, no longer knowing how to open himself to other people except by experiencing them through the lenses of his own egocentrism.

Samadeva Gestural Euphony is able to avoid these dangers by also integrating movements and active, conscious thought. The dynamic exercises, practiced standing or sitting down, allow the participant to go beyond the stage of dream consciousness associated with the horizontal position; he must become conscious of his physical environment, which is integrated into the exercises in such a way that he is directly confronted with it. It is understood that each person has his own particularities, pace of work, limits, psychological problems, and so on.

the dynamic exercises and active attention

Samadeva Gestural Euphony is addressed to the man and woman who, assuming the vertical position after the Old Testament Fall, is endowed with the first spark of consciousness, of a psychological "I", and clothed in a physical body. This body was, at first, much subtler than it is today, but forces of hardening and densification subsequently introduced themselves, with the result that man became more and more interested in material substances and forces, leading to a premature hardening and densification of his body. Impressions, emotions, and thoughts inscribed themselves to a greater extent on this body and, as a

the path of the human soul through time and the evolution of worlds result, man descended much too deeply into the world of materiality. The physical body thus progressively became as we know it today, composed of a skeleton, muscles, tendons, nerves, and covered with skin. It is to this body, born of our confrontation with matter and life on earth, that the exercises—promoting as they do our joint flexibility, muscle extension, and emotional and intellectual relaxation—are addressed. Through these exercises, the participant rediscovers physical movements and gestures that are more effective and appropriate to the conditions of his everyday life; this is achieved by attaining optimal muscle tone with minimal effort, liberating the psyche of its tensions in the process.

Samadeva Gestural Euphony brings a new harmony to all of the vital and psychic processes connected to the body

Samadeva Gestural Euphony thus works on the one hand through relaxation, in which the participant is placed in a state of conscious dreaming, and on the other through dynamic exercises addressed to incarnate man, whose physical body must become an effective tool in the face of the demands of life on earth, perfectly adapted to his emotional and intellectual functioning. Through a newly acquired consciousness of the body and its connections to the psyche, and through a rediscovery of spontaneous movements that do not hinder the organic functions, Samadeva Gestural Euphony creates a bridge between the expansive forces present in the unconscious and the hardening, densifying forces also present in man. It brings a new harmony to all the vital and psychic processes of the body, allowing the participant to liberate and manifest his possibilities of development and creativity. Since this con-

a bridge between the expansive forces of the unconscious and the hardening, densifying forces present in man

sciousness is acquired by refining the body's sensations, it is certainly of interest to examine the senses concerned. They are twelve in number, although science currently recognizes only the five most apparent among them.

In addition to the five senses of touch, sight, hearing, smell, and taste, Samadeva Gestural Euphony includes the seven senses that connect man to his mind and psyche:

- The sense of heat, not the same as the sense of touch, as it involves another quality different from the quality that allows us to distinguish, for example, between smooth and rough.

- The sense of balance, which allows us to perceive our position in space.

- The sense of movement, allowing us, through the activity of our muscles and limbs in the external world, to perceive whether we are moving or at rest.

- The sense of life, allowing us to enter into the depths of our organism, giving us information about the general vital state of our organs and the harmonious functioning of our body's vital processes.

- The sense of speech, as the sense of hearing does not suffice for recognizing external sounds as human speech.

- The sense of thought, which allows us to understand the thought contained in a fragment of speech.

in addition to the five usual senses, Samadeva Gestural Euphony includes the seven senses that connect man to his mind and psyche

- The sense of "I," which enables us to perceive the "I" of other people.

Our work includes all the senses in order to connect physical man to his mind and psyche and, beyond these, to the world and people around him.

the fundamental role of consciousness of the body

We can understand the fundamental role played by consciousness of the body, for it brings us back to man's first experience of matter during the distant epoch of the "Fall," when he parted from his initial obscure consciousness and abandoned the horizontal position of the animal, voluntarily straightening himself into the vertical position. He was now able to perceive himself independently of his environment, as a distinct entity, as a spirit occupying a body isolated in space but nonetheless perfectly connected to it.

His contact with material realities, as well as his body's impenetrability, confronted man with forces that provided a necessary resistance for his spiritual activity; now the spirit could return to itself, it could be thought and perceived in the same way as light in a mirror. The body therefore serves as a reflecting apparatus that gives rise to consciousness, allowing the "I" to see itself from the outside, to be "reflected" on like someone who "is" and feels that he "is." This desire to "be" already manifests itself in the vertical position acquired by man, triumphing over the force of gravity, a position connecting the higher with the lower, cosmic with terrestrial forces.

the body: a mirror that gives rise to consciousness

This experience, in which the spirit ceases to be blended with the cosmos, isolating itself in a physical body, evolved slowly, reaching a decisive turning point at the Renaissance. During this epoch, man lost the living feeling that he belongs to the cosmos. Feeling himself as a unique individual is a necessary experience, but it deprives him of the protection of the gods and places him face to face with his own freedom; he is cut off from the spiritual world and from nature, which no longer appear inhabited by elementary forces, becoming instead inert, mineral, "inanimate."

Through the practice of Samadeva Gestural Euphony, the relationship between body and psyche changes once again. The participant no longer feels himself as a being isolated in his body, but acquires a further dimension of relationship with other people and the surrounding world. This can bring him into contact with a spiritual reality in himself, and possibly with a more universal, unifying consciousness. The latter may culminate in a mystical experience.

The experience of having a body and "being a body" thus not only confronts the participant with his own feelings and unconscious, but also integrates the part of his being directed toward the spiritual world, his Higher "I," whose psychological "I" is but a feeble reflection that does not reveal its essence. When we become conscious of our body, this can lead us to the realization that we are, as it were, a hieroglyph of the cosmos, a microcosm born of the macrocosm. We can thus understand today's fascination with the body, our determination to dissect it, to search for psycho-physiological reflexes, our desire to unveil the mystery of its composition and functioning. We also find

recognize oneself as a
hieroglyph of the cosmos

the reason behind our infatuation with the body, to which we devote more and more of our time, money, and attention. The experience of the body that we propose allows us not only to establish the connection between body and psyche, but to rediscover the deep connection between body and spirit.

rediscover the deep connection between body and spirit

The mind is what fundamentally makes this connection possible, since the mind alone can lead us to a clear consciousness of our body and of ourselves. It is the mind that reestablishes order among all the soul impressions resurfacing from the depths, "recognizing" and "understanding" them, that is to say, genuinely making them our own, so that we are born anew with them. We can thus make a new connection between, on the one hand, the hidden desires of our metabolism and our unconscious, and on the other, the clear, free will issuing from our reflection, emerging from our higher psyche. We must have the courage to descend into the depths of our body in order to cast light not only upon our repressed emotions, but above all upon the slumbering seeds of will inside us, identifying them through our clear and living thought, and integrating them into our free and responsible being.

a work of harmonization and liberation

This is the path proposed by the exercises of Samadeva Gestural Euphony, with the aim of elevating and organizing everything that rises up from the depths of our unconscious and liberating it from its conditioning, mechanisms, and materiality. It is thus, from both a physical and mental point of view, a work of harmonization and liberation.

SAMADEVA AND QUANTUM PHYSICS: FROM SCIENCE TO WISDOM

Idris Lahore

the transcendence of the
ego through liberating and
creative inner development

The psychology of Samadeva Gestural Euphony can be counted among the "transpersonal psychologies" that teach the transcendence of the ego, not in the sense of a pathological annihilation, but of a liberating and creative inner development.

Beyond its corporal techniques, Samadeva Gestural Euphony can lead the participant who so desires to a deeper understanding than in the ordinary approach, limited as it is to the perception of appearances and unable to pierce to the substance, the essence of things.

experiencing a previously
unknown dimension of reality

Through the psycho-corporal techniques and the experiences they awaken, it is possible for us to experience a previously unknown dimension of reality. This is not a matter of mystical delirium, but a possibility of experience transcending the limits of sensory perception, without in any way denying the necessary adaptation of material man to the material world; the transcendence of sensory limitations goes hand-in-hand with the immanent and inclusive dimension that characterizes a mind liberated from conditioning.

This can of course be discussed alongside the experiments made by physicists J. A. Wheeler or F. A. Popp, demonstrating that photons possess a certain conscious, intelligent energy capable of entering into spiritual interaction with man's own consciousness and intelligence. And we may continue on to the researches of the no less famous physicist David Bohm, friend of the Hindu sage Krishnamurti, or the work of semanticist G. Tiry.

The essential principle of physics at the end of the twentieth century and beginning of the third millennium is that the universe is an undivided biological entity in which matter, composed of particles, is alive, possessing a consciousness and intelligence of which the consciousness and intelligence of man are only a manifestation. Scientific knowledge here joins the spiritual teachings of the great sages, of Aurobindo, Gurdjieff, Steiner, Krishnamurti or, more recently, Selim Aïssel.

the universe has a consciousness and an intelligence

The conscious and conscientious practice of Samadeva Gestural Euphony can lead us to this meeting point, to the understanding, or rather intuition of Reality that goes beyond the capacities of the brain alone, encompassing man in all of his physical, emotional, and intellectual dimensions.

intuition of Reality that goes beyond the capacities of the brain alone

This Reality corresponds to the Absolute or Numinous of the spiritualists, the Divine of the religious, and finally to the ultimate reality of the scientist when he explains to us the "subquantic mechanism of virtual transitions," proving that a place exists where material space becomes memory and time becomes eternity.

a place exists where material space becomes memory and time becomes eternity

attaining to a unifying
intuition of our being and
that of the world, and to the
complete identicalness of
their essences

The participant may thus, if he wishes, attain to a unifying vision of his own being and that of the world, and to the complete identicalness of their essences, in the same manner that a David Bohm or Rupert Sheldrake attain to a holistic vision of the universe through their scientific work.

Wisdom, that practical Gnosis, is no longer the privilege of a few ascetics or monks withdrawn from the world, but becomes a possibility for scientific research or for daily psycho-corporal practice like that taught in the context of Samadeva Gestural Euphony. These two paths lead to a perfect integration of man, not only with his family, social, or professional environment, but also of his most superficial ego with its profound essence, and beyond it, to the essence of the universe. We are thus dealing with genuine practices of Realization and Awakening.

genuine practices of
Realization and Awakening

THE HEALING TECHNIQUES OF THE DERVISHES

Idris Lahore

T he search for immortality: is this not one of humanity's oldest dreams? Philosophers have thought about
it for ages, religions promise it after death, Taoists practice
exercises for longevity, alchemists prepare the elixir of
long life, and scientists, while denying its existence,
attempt to freeze the body in order to one day bring it back
to life. Where is the truth in all this? How much is legend
and how much reality?

The Origin of Samadeva

I would like to tell you the story of how the search for
immortality led me to Kafiristan, where I met Pir Kejttep
Ancari. He was the spiritual master, the Sheikh of a dervish
brotherhood said to be descended from the Magi of the
Orient. Three of them had followed the star to the cradle
of Bethlehem.

Doctors and priests, healers and magicians, they used
trance and hypnosis, plants and poisons, physical and respiratory exercises, energetic techniques and what are
today known as systemic therapies. Some of them are still
alive today; their secrets, jealously guarded, are passed on
in the brotherhood from master to pupil, from soul to soul.

Their knowledge and practices are the vestiges of the medicine which flourished in the great Arab universities of the Middle Ages, from the Middle East to the West, from Gondichapur to Toledo. These dervishes are known as the Sarmans; they are said to be the Masters of Time and to possess the secrets of immortality. During the time I spent with Pir Kejttep Ancari, he taught me, among other things, the healing techniques of the dervishes. I was the first and shall remain the only Westerner to receive the Initiation from him. He transmitted to me the Baraka that I may in turn transmit it to the West. When he spoke to me for the first time, I recalled the words of Padmasambhava, another great sage who belonged to the Tibetan Buddhist tradition : "When the iron birds fly, the Dharma shall come to the West." This prophecy is being fulfilled in our time.

Received into the monastery into which the old Master had retired, among carefully chosen disciples and in the greatest secrecy, I began a training considered to be the most esoteric. In other books I have presented certain dervish techniques in the form taught me by the Master, and in the form he authorized me to reveal.

My education was of the mind, heart, and body. The goal of this extremely rigorous training was to develop in students a complete mastery of the different constituents of their being: intellectual, emotional, and physical. These techniques lead to the mastery of the thoughts, the purification of the feelings and emotions, and finally, as in certain forms of yoga, to a conscious use of the functions connected to the physical centers: sexual energy in the sexual center; breathing, blood circulation, assimilation of food, and hormonal secretions in the instinctive center; and external movements and attitudes in the moving center. The purpose of this esoteric training was, to cite the words of the Tradition, to transform ordinary man into "perfected man."

My theoretical and practical studies were followed by trials (today they would be called tests or examinations) revealing the level the student had attained. According to the Tradition, thirty-three years (4 times 8, plus 1 year) are necessary to attain complete mastery of the "art of immortality" of the body and the soul. The Hakim—as these healers of body and soul are known—made me think at once of the Essene brotherhoods, the healers from the time of Jesus of Nazareth, who were also known as Therapeuts. My studies of Greek reminded me that in the past, the word "therapy" meant "sacred service."

During the night from Thursday evening to Friday morning, the monastery received dozens of visitors with various illnesses, some of them from very distant countries; during my time there, I saw Kafiristani peasants, Hindu princes, Chinese and Russian politicians, Iranian imams and dignitaries, and a Saudi oil magnate. All were suffering from illnesses said to be incurable.

The Pir Hakim, *pir* meaning old—in the East at the time, old age was still synonymous with wisdom—the Master whose disciple I had become, was surrounded by nine other healers, and they first received the sick in a large hall, the white walls illuminated by the gentle light emanating from oil lamps. On the floor could be seen the symbol known by initiates as "the sign of God on earth," the enneagram. One of the nine Hakim stood at each point of the enneagram. The Master was seated on a white sheepskin within the central triangle. Each visitor was led to him by an assistant. After greeting him with the greatest respect and placing their gifts at his feet, the patients sat on their heels, facing the Master who, one by one, placed their hands in his own and breathed upon their foreheads according to an ancient ritual known as Tcheff-Hu-Hakim (the breath of the healer of God). After this he whispered some words into the patient's ear intended to initiate the process of healing. The patient was then instructed to stand and was led to one of the nine other Hakim, as indicated by the Master. The Hakim repeated the Master's gestures, then sang the healing words together with the patient until he was certain that he had learned them by heart. He then held his hand and pressed it several consecutive times with his thumb, after which he placed two fingers on other parts of his body, asking the patient to inhale and exhale deeply. Thanks to my studies of Chinese medicine, I recognized that the zones being treated, called Lataif or Taj by the dervishes, corresponded in each case to different acupuncture points. In contrast to Chinese medicine, the Hakim did not insert any needles on these points, applying instead a pressure with his fingers, tapping them, or breathing upon them, asking the patient at the same time to concentrate on his illness or problem. These techniques were intended to harmonize the circulation of the energies Nafa in the patient's body, heart, and mind, after which he was shown a movement or gesture that he was to practice regularly once he had returned home. These exercises were called "Arkanas." The patient was then led to the surrounding wall, where he seated himself, still repeating the words he had received in a low voice. The bed-ridden were carried to the Master by the assistants, then stretched out beside the same walls. So the hall was filled with the low murmur of various melodies, yet never resulting in the cacophony one might have expected; on the contrary, during the course of the night I had the growing impression of an immense presence, of an immense, yet gentle force growing continually stronger. It was as if everything had become at once purer, calmer, denser—the air, the light, the murmur of the voices, and even the time that was passing.

After a time several of the patients would fall asleep, but the Hakim, after the sick had all been seated or stretched out along the walls, continued to recite and quietly chant the sacred verses, regularly applying pressures to the points on their own bodies that corresponded to the points that had been used for the patients. This continued until sunrise. After all of the visitors had, without exception, fallen asleep, they were woken by the Hakim. They placed their hands upon the patients' shoulders and whispered a few words into their ears; most of them seemed to be emerging from a very deep sleep, and I myself had the impression of being in one of the temples of sleep and healing of Greek antiquity, as if I had traveled back in time.

All of the sick people were in a tranquil state, and even to see the formerly bed-ridden standing up and walking around seemed normal, although of course this was extraordinary. Joyful serenity and profound gratitude illuminated the faces of those present. Not everyone had been healed yet, or healed entirely, but each visitor seemed to have been visited by an angel during the course of the night, an angel who had, at the least, granted him the gift of the joy of living. And perhaps, for those who had not yet been healed, this was the beginning of a process of healing that would last several days or several months. In any case this is what my Master explained to me.

The assistants returned to lead the sick to another room, where they were served a meal before being brought back to the doors of the monastery, after giving them the customary warnings: to never and under no pretext whatsoever speak of the methods used by the Hakim, or else their illness would return immediately, this time rendered incurable. They were also informed that the powers of healing—the Baraka—that they had received acted over the course of several days and perhaps even several months, and that through them, they were connected to the living Master, Pir Kejttep Ancari, to his Master, to his Master's Master, and through them to the succession of all Masters (Silsilla) back to Adam at the beginning of time and, through Adam, to God Himself.

In spite of these indications, no religious demand was made of the visitor; he did not even have to be a believer. This was in marked contrast to the numerous religious or spiritual healing techniques which demand conversion as the price of health—in this case, no propaganda. Just before taking leave of the patients, the Hakim reminded them of the healing words and showed them the pressure points one last time, giving them, as it were, a final therapeutic prescription. To certain others, they showed a posture that was to be adopted or a movement to be made, which was to accompany the recitation or chanting of the words.

My Master, shortly before my departure from the monastery, spoke to me thus: "Gradually translate and transcribe the songs and words that I whisper into the ears of the sick and that they sing themselves afterward. You will teach them to one of your pupils, whom you will initiate yourself into their understanding. You will observe, as I have taught you, the effects of reading, reciting, and singing them on the mind, heart, and body; above all, you will observe their effect on the soul and spiritual essence of man. You will see that each of these verses is a form of medicine. Do the same for the Arkana movements. For certain illnesses, these exercises will be more effective than medicinal plants and mineral remedies, more effective even than most remedies invented by man. Know that those who practice these Arkanas and recite or sing these verses, especially those who understand and love them, will make a great step toward attaining immortality. They are the elixir of eternal youth."

Something even stranger and more extraordinary could be witnessed on Monday evenings, continuing over the course of the entire night until the following morning. This was called the "night of reconciliation with the ancestors," during which, according to the Hakim, the souls of the ancestors could find peace once again. Before explaining the profound meaning behind this technique, I will simply describe what I saw when I participated for the first time in this mysterious night of reconciliation.

A gentle light emanating from oil lamps once again illuminated the large hall with its white walls, the ground covered this time with thick carpets leaving open only the circle of the enneagram. Nine Hakim were seated around the enneagram; as for the Master, he was seated outside the circle on a low table serving as a platform. Men, women, and even children were packed together along the entire length of the walls, perhaps a hundred in all, belonging visibly to very different social classes. Beside the women clothed in chadors sat others who, in their silk attire, could have been princesses out of the Arabian Nights; peasants in their heavy wool coats were seated next to men in Western dress, with their white shirts, jackets, and ties.

The men and most of the women were seated in silence and meditative presence, as if reflecting the immobility and silence of the nine Hakim around the circle. Even the children seemed to be won over by this atmosphere of peace, and the simple smile and attention of their mother seemed to suffice for their needs.

Suddenly, the Master's firm voice resounds in the silence, like a question. A few moments pass, and all eyes are fixed upon him. One man who had been seated along the wall rises with a serious expression, looks at the Master, bows toward him with respect, then looks at him once more. The Master signals for him to advance. After arriving in front of him, he bows once again, and the Master asks him to take a seat beside him upon the platform. A short dialogue ensues, which seems to be the evocation of a problem. The Master signals for the man to stand up. He enters the circle and bows successively before six of the nine Hakim seated around the circumference of the enneagram. The six Hakim rise as if they had been chosen. The man looks toward the Master, who makes another sign accompanied by a few words. The man then positions himself behind the first of the six Hakim, placing the palms of his hands on his shoulders, and pushes him toward the center of the circle, after which he stops suddenly. The man looks again at the Master, who points to a second Hakim, and the same scenario is repeated: the man positions himself behind the Hakim, places both his hands on his upper back, and pushes him toward another point on the circle. He does the same with the four other Hakim he had asked to stand. The Master summons him once again to take a seat beside him. The Hakim are now standing in the circle of the enneagram; one is staring at the ground, another is looking toward the outside, three others are looking at each other, and the last is covering his eyes with his hands. Suddenly, I hear the Master exclaim with a powerful voice, "Allah Hu!", meaning "the breath of God." Now the most striking thing happens: one of the dervishes immediately steps out of the circle and walks out of the great white hall; another collapses to the ground and lies outstretched on his back, like a dead person; the one who had placed his hands over his eyes advances up to the limit of the circle, and turning his back to the scene, looks in a completely different direction. The two who had been standing close to each other walk toward the one lying upon the ground and look at him, apparently with great sadness. This all happens as in a slow-motion film, and I have the impression that the space has become denser. None of the onlookers moves, not even the children; they all seem to be holding their breath. Everyone seems spellbound until, suddenly, as if obeying one and the same signal, three women who had been seated among the crowd rise from their places and, weeping, throw themselves at the Hakim who seems to be representing a dead person. One of them grasps his feet, another takes hold of his hand, and the third, her face buried in her hands, bends over his head. At the same time, next to the impassable Master, I see the man pull a large cloth out of his pocket and use it as a handkerchief to dry his eyes, overcome by a strong emotion before the spectacle of which he is at the origin. For a few minutes, as if the time were frozen, all of the protagonists in the circle continue their own movement, until the voice of the Master resounds once again: "Allah Hu!" he exclaims, rising from his seat. He walks toward the inside of the circle, signals for all of those kneeling or lying on the ground, one by one, to stand up, straightens the ones who are bent over, calls back the Hakim who had left the hall, and gathers them all together into a circle in which the protagonists from the scene I have just described are to hold each other's hands. After they have been gathered together, the Master, in the middle of the inner circle, pronounces a word, and everyone in the circle looks toward the ground, chanting together with him, "Allah Hu, Allah Hu, Allah Hu"; their faces become illuminated with an inner light, as if each of them were suddenly filled with a deep joy. Indeed, they start looking at each other, now smiling, as if a problem had been resolved. The Master then makes a gesture toward the man who had been seated beside him, inviting him to take the place of one of the Hakim, who returns to his seat on one of the points of the enneagram. The man, still visibly moved, enters the circle, and he, too, is overcome by this energy of joy, transforming his emotion; his face lights up and his sadness gives way to a shining countenance. The Master's voice resounds once again. Everyone is silent, and making a sign, he opens the circle. Each person returns to his place—the Hakim to the circumference of the enneagram, the three women alongside the wall, and the man beside the Master, who speaks to him a few more words. The man then bows before the Master, takes his hand in his own, kisses it, and lifts it to his forehead while the Master, with a gesture full of love, places his other hand upon his head; then pressing his shoulders lightly, he raises him up, and signals for him to return to his place alongside the wall. After the man has seated himself, another man stands up, bows, and walks toward the Master. The same type of scenario begins again and is repeated many times over the course of the night;

each time a man or woman chooses several of the nine Hakim from the circumference of the enneagram, and each time different protagonists stand up from among the crowd seated along the walls in order to participate in the scene. During the course of the night, some people fall asleep, others wake up, but as for myself, I am so spellbound by what is taking place before my eyes that I do not even notice the passing of the night. In the early morning, the Master rises and walks out of the hall, accompanied by the nine Hakim, and the students of the monastery remain until the men, women, and children have all left the premises.

The explanation of what had happened at first seemed to me even more extraordinary than what I had seen. Since then, I know that there is nothing extraordinary about it, and that it is nothing more than the manifestation of completely natural faculties that every person possesses, provided he or she allows them to be expressed in certain conditions.

The Master explained to me what I had seen and what I would later present to my students as "euphonic representations of the movements of the soul," in the context of Systemic Samadeva, variants of which are known to Westerners as psychodramas and family therapies or constellations, one of the sources of which I had obviously witnessed. This was also the fundamental component of theatre at the time of Greek antiquity.

The Monastery of Immortality, said to have existed since the beginning of time, is surrounded by a wealth of mysterious legends. It is said, for example, that only men and women can find it whose heart and intentions are pure. For the others it is completely inaccessible, even if they hold the map in their very hands. It is also said that over the course of every nine years, it disappears twice, along with all of its inhabitants, for two years, only to reappear again as if out of nowhere, or from another world.

Without betraying the secrets entrusted to me that I cannot reveal except to those following a path of initiation, I have nevertheless been permitted to relate what I saw during my first visit to the Monastery of Immortality. It was the very first time I visited the man who was said to be one of the living Masters of Wisdom. I will not mention all of the obstacles I had to surmount in order to arrive at the foot of the mountain where the Monastery was to be found.

Standing before the entrance, I ring the bell. After a few moments the door opens and a young man of about thirty appears, of rare beauty. Whether he is a servant or prince, I cannot say. After I introduce myself, he leads me through several long corridors to my room and tells me that I can wash up and have a short rest. A bowl of fruit and a steaming teapot and cup are sitting on the table. Hardly an hour has passed before he returns, leading me through the premises and showing me everything I would need to be familiar with. The style is medieval: there are stone walls, woodcuts, and Oriental tapestries. The atmosphere of the rooms is mysterious, yet at the same time warm and welcoming. During the course of the visit, we meet several different people; none of them are presented to me, but they all greet me with a smile. Each makes the same impression on me of a certain detached elegance, at the same time warm and welcoming, that I find in my guide.

He finally leads me to another wing of the building in which there are no private rooms. He explains that we are passing through the study and work halls. The first is the same room I have described above, the hall in which the sick are received; at the moment it is empty. Then, after opening some heavy doors, I can hear music and singing, or rather declaimed words, resonating from the end of the corridor, and as we approach the next hall, the music becomes louder and louder. It is another large hall; in it about a dozen musicians are seated in a circle, playing melodies that I cannot place in any category known to me, neither Eastern nor Western. But the impression is so strong that the first melody I hear remains in my memory to this day. We pass through the hall without the musicians taking the slightest notice of us.

In the adjoining halls, about a dozen people are practicing movements and dances of a special nature that I have never seen before. Later my instructors would teach me these movements, actually therapeutic gymnastics, as well as sacred dances and music. These physical exercises form the basis of the Arkanas of Samadeva Gestural Euphony.

Further halls are occupied by calligraphers, painters, and sculptors, all working in the utmost silence. Then we pass through two rooms resembling the laboratories of a chemist, or rather of an alchemist of the Middle Ages, with vials, test tubes, and several jars apparently containing plants and various kinds of liquids. In these rooms I would later be initiated into the art of "healing fragrances," the therapeutic use of certain herbal essences and incense.

Finally we come to a large door leading into an inner garden, in the midst of which is a fountain. My guide, of whose name I am still ignorant, informs me, "The Master will receive you early this evening. Until then, you are free to walk through the premises, have a rest, or take part in the various activities in the study and work halls. If you need my help, you will find me." Then, after another enigmatic smile, he leaves me alone before the fountain.

The sound of the water reminds me of Zarathustra's words, "And my soul also is a bubbling fountain." Yes, I have only been here for a few hours and my soul is already full of impressions, each one of them as rich as the next.

Is it the activities I witnessed or the Monastery's unusual atmosphere? Everything here appears at once so simple and yet sacred, a feeling utterly new to me and yet somehow familiar, as if I already knew this place, these people, these activities, as if an old and deeply buried memory had resurfaced to my consciousness. Nonetheless, I am here for the first time in my life—or should I rather say, in this life?

My guide returns to lead me about thirty meters along a path running outside the Monastery, to a house apparently lying in ruins; but one of the rooms is inhabitable, and this is where the Master resides. We walk around the little building, and I discern a silhouette in the distance, clothed in white. It is Pir Kejttep Ancari. We walk together towards him, or rather I have the impression that my guide is walking beside me, whereas in fact, with the greatest discretion, he has withdrawn without my noticing and I am suddenly left alone with the Master. His white hair is concealed by a turban. When I perceive the smile upon his lips, in the middle of his long white beard, I realize that I am in the presence of a man whose entire being radiates beauty and love. In spite of his great age—he is said to be more than 144 years old—his forehead has not a single wrinkle, and his eyes are so lucid, despite their dark color, that they could be the eyes of an eagle gazing into the most profound depths of your being. This look, a look of understanding and intelligence, together with his welcoming smile, reassure me entirely: a man like this knows what he is doing.

He receives me into his dwelling. His first words are an invitation to walk with him through the forest. The Monastery is located just below the forest, and we have hardly advanced three hundred meters when we encounter a tiger on the path. I sense fear and even terror arising within me. The Master takes a firm hold of my hand, and I am immediately filled with the greatest peace. The tiger approaches, calmly, within a few paces of us, then disappears into the bushes just as calmly. Pir Kejttep Ancari tells me, "He and I are completely free of fear. That is why we can both walk calmly through the forest." I would not understand this event until much later, and for a long time I could not say whether it was a dream or reality.

Our conversation lasts an hour, and I leave his dwelling with the certainty that I have met not only a remarkable man, but also a man who, in his everyday life, incarnates the highest spiritual principles, a man who drinks from the wellspring of knowledge and being, of wisdom and of life.

But an even more extraordinary legend is told about Pir Kejttep Ancari. He is said to be the Kidhr, considered by the mystics of many religions to be the eternal man. He is said to be the prophet Elijah at the origin of all spiritualities. It was he who was said to have initiated Mohammed and Moses even before the latter ascended Mount Sinai. Considered to be the Hidden Master, he reveals himself in an individual way to each spiritual seeker during the course of his path of initiation. Some people say that he is always incarnated and that every seeker meets him at least once during the course of his life.

The nomads of the desert tell his marvellous story. For them, he is not only the patron saint of travelers, thieves, and merchants, but above all incarnates divine providence. Whoever encounters him must never ask him any questions, but must follow his counsel, as extravagant as it may seem, since the Kidhr always indicates the path of truth, health, and happiness behind appearances that can sometimes be absurd. Then, having rendered his service, he vanishes from sight.

According to some, he is the son of Adam himself and saved the body of his father during the Flood. He is said to have been born in a cave. Sometimes he is identified with Saint George or the Archangel Michael slaying the dragon. He is also held to be the Hermes Trismegistus of the alchemists. He is said to have attained to the wellspring of life, from which he has drunk and in which he has bathed, thus attaining immortality. It is he who knows the secret of eternal youth.

Legend or reality? This is all I have been permitted to relate publicly. It is now my wish for the reader to find hope, health, and harmony through what I have been given and allowed to pass on.

THE NINE BRANCHES
OF SAMADEVA

Idris Lahore

The nine branches of Samadeva are an approach that truly takes into account all the constituents of man as well as his spiritual dimension. It also takes into account his relationship with the people around him and with nature. In this chapter we will present in summary these nine branches, each of which may be discovered at the Free University of Samadeva located in Alsace, France, and particularly during its annual congress.

Free University of Samadeva

The first branch includes Samadeva Gestural Euphony and the Euphonic Techniques of Relaxation.

First Branch

Samadeva Gestural Euphony

• Samadeva Gestural Euphony is the ne plus ultra of psycho-corporal methods. The method consists of movements and postures practiced to the accompaniment of music specially created for the purpose. It unites oriental approaches resembling tai chi chuan, qi gong, and yoga, with other, more Western approaches, such as eurhythmy, stretching, and relaxation. Inspired by the most ancient traditions, it is perfectly adapted to the needs and values of the men and women of today, with their more hurried and more sedentary lifestyle. In this book, we have presented to you its most fundamental component, the seven major Arkanas.

- The Euphonic Techniques of Relaxation (ETR) are an answer to stress and pain. Their source dates back millennia, drawing upon the knowledge of ancient therapeutic traditions. The basic techniques involve attention to ourselves through our body, emotions, and thoughts. They are allied to specific breathing techniques performed standing, seated, or lying down, in addition to slow or dynamic movements. The Euphonic Techniques of Relaxation are of particular interest to people suffering from the effects of stress, chronic troubles, and pain. They also make possible an improvement in intellectual, bodily, and athletic performance.

Euphonic Techniques of Relaxation (E.T.R.)

The Articular Treatments permit a gentle correction of problems in the joints and vertebral column. This is achieved by means of simple techniques. The back and limbs reacquire their flexibility, tone, and agility, and an improved bodily and nervous equilibrium result.

*Second Branch
Articular Treatments*

The method includes:

- Articular Adjustments and Auto-Adjustments: simple movements permitting the elimination of many forms of pain, of an inflammatory, muscular, or articular origin, resulting from micro- or subluxations.

Articular Adjustments and Auto-Adjustments

- The Arkanas of revitalization and dynamization.

- Several types of massage, as well as Euphonic and Energetic Touch, combining the most modern techniques with traditional techniques of the East and West, and permitting relaxation, greater vitality, the resolution

Euphonic Energetic Touch

of psychological tensions, and a free circulation of the energies.

The techniques include, among others, the Energetic Touch for the face; the activation of the energetic pathways, Silsilla, or meridians in the limbs, which are massaged lightly, releasing blockages; the gentle, rhythmic, and energizing Hakim Euphonic Touch for the back, which has an action on the entire body, internal organs, and psyche, liberating emotional, physical, and energetic tensions.

Third Branch Meridian Energetic Techniques (M.E.T.)

The Meridian Energetic Techniques unite the knowledge of Chinese, Ayurvedic, Yunnani, and Dervish medicine, all of which recognize the presence of energetic and informatic systems in man. Troubles and illnesses are considered to be disruptions in the circulation of energy and information; these techniques of energetic harmonization, rebalancing the circulation of energy and readjusting the flow of information, have a more rapid and profound effect than the majority of other therapeutic techniques.

Fourth Branch Psychology of the Enneagram

The Psychology of the Enneagram permits us to better know ourselves and better know other people, and thus to better live and work together. With the Enneagram, we learn that people function according to nine different types, conforming to mechanisms specific to their "type," and revealing problem areas that the Psychology of the Enneagram enables us to resolve.

Fifth Branch Essential Psychology

The Essential Psychology is one of the most profound transpersonal approaches. Going beyond the psychological observation of man's functioning, it provides the means for

181

overcoming the ego, with the aim of realizing one's Essence, what is highest in oneself.

Alchemical or Spagyric Energetic Medicine, on a mineral and plant basis, dates from the dawn of time and has been adapted to the conditions of our day.

Sixth Branch
Alchemical or Spagyric
Energetic Medicine

This branch associates the most recent research in dietetics and nutrition with the traditional dietetic approach of the dervishes, adapted to the men and women of today.

Seventh Branch
Dietetics and Nutrition

Art, structures, and radiations consists of an accumulation of knowledge resembling Chinese feng shui or Indian vastu. This branch of Samadeva involves the study of the influence of art, structures, forms, and radiations (telluric radiation, for example) on our health.

Eighth Branch
Art, structures, and radiations

A very ancient art, Systemic Samadeva, also called "euphonic representations of the movements of the soul," resembles the more well-known forms of transgenerational therapies and other family constellations.

Systemic Samadeva is a form of therapeutic work done in the context of a group, with the goal of helping a person and, through him or her, all the people with whom he or she is in relationship. It permits us to find our just place as we reconcile ourselves with the painful elements of our past, acquiring the necessary strength to accept or face the present.

Ninth Branch
Systemic Samadeva of
"Euphonic Representations
of the Movements
of the Soul"

Carried out silently, gently, and with infinite respect, this therapeutic work involves the "movement of the soul," which often manifests itself through very slow gestures that are beyond any subjective interpretation.

THE AUTHORS

IDRIS LAHORE has been immersed in both Eastern and Western traditions and cultures since his childhood. Over the course of his extensive travels and studies throughout the world, he acquired a profound knowledge of these traditions and a subtle understanding of the human psyche. A painter, poet, and prolific author, Idris Lahore is also a great observer and discoverer. We recall Goethe, discoverer of the Sufi poets; today we can appreciate the many works of Idris Lahore which, with pertinence and precision, describe the therapeutic art of the dervishes, Samadeva, an essential art of healing, health, and harmony.

ENNEA TESS GRIFFITH has practiced numerous psycho-corporal techniques since her earliest youth, including such eastern techniques as yoga, tai chi chuan, qi gong, and Samadeva Gestural Euphony as well as western techniques such as stretching, eurhythmy, and Bothmer gymnastics. Trained in the healing techniques of the dervishes by Idris Lahore for several years, Ennea Tess Griffith has been working to make the ancient knowledge and practical methods of the dervishes accessible to Westerners. With Idris Lahore, she developed the nine branches of Samadeva taught at the Free University of Samadeva, of which she is the founder, directing many of the university's seminars and courses. She teaches several introductory and advanced courses, particularly in Samadeva Gestural Euphony, Zhi Neng Qi Gong, and Meridian Energetic Techniques.

EMMA THYLOCH was trained by Idris Lahore in the psycho-corporal techniques of the dervishes, which she has taught for ten years. Cofounder of the Free University of Samadeva, she teaches several courses and seminars in Samadeva Gestural Euphony, Nadi Yoga, and Gurdjieff Dances and Movements. In addition, she organizes classes and workshops throughout Europe. In the context of one of the nine branches of Samadeva, Emma Thyloch also teaches training courses in Euphonic and Energetic Massage.

To LEARN MORE about Dervish Yoga (Samadeva Gestural Euphony), and for information on courses and seminars offered for both beginners and professionals, please contact:

FREE UNIVERSITY OF SAMADEVA
LE CLOS ERMITAGE
34 Rue du Wittertalhof • 67140 le Hohwald • France
PH: 0033 (0)388 08 31 31
email: info@libre-universite-samadeva.com
www.libre-universite-samadeva.com
English-language inquiries: 0033 (0)388 08 51 36

A CD and DVD have been specially created for the practice of the seven major Arkanas, and is available through the Free University of Samadeva.